1,000+ Barbara O'Neill Natural Herbal Remedies

Natural Remedies for All Kinds of Aliments and Health Conditions

Aveline Clarke

ISBN 978-1-7637505-0-0 (Paperback)

ISBN 978-1-7637505-1-7 (Hardcover)

Cover Design by Rgraphic

It includes assets from Pixabay & Freepik

Published by Boundless Stories

Written by Aveline Clarke

Edited by Amanda Clarke

First Edition (2024)

YOUR EXCLUSIVE GIFTS

As a gesture of appreciation for your support, I've included a few free gifts—just for you.

You can access these by scanning the QR code at the end of the book, thoughtfully kept there to ensure it remains exclusive for my cherished readers.

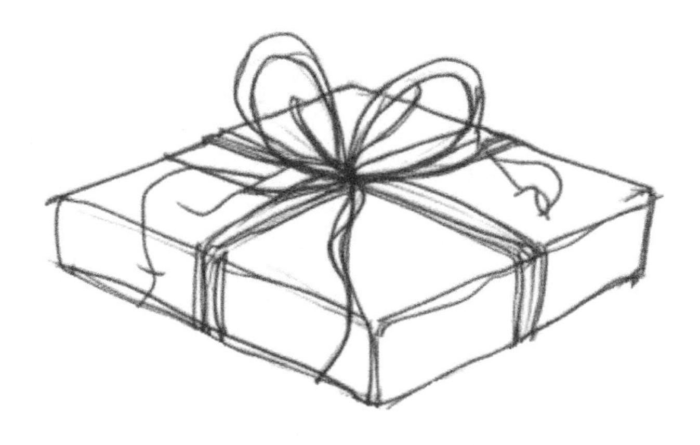

Along with your gifts, you'll get access to exclusive giveaways, special offers, and insightful tips curated just for you.

That said, enjoy the read—and thank you for joining me on this journey!

Aveline Clarke

Table of Contents

Disclaimer

While Barbara O'Neill's teachings profoundly inspired the creation of this book, it isn't officially connected to or endorsed by her. Her teachings are used for educational purposes and to provide insight into the use of herbal and folk remedies identified by the author. Neither Barbara O'Neill nor her affiliates have explicitly approved the views presented in this book.

While not a medical professional, the author has taken the time to provide accurate and safe information. However, they cannot be held responsible for interpretations of subject material, omissions, or possible errors that may come to light with the continual research in the field of herbal remedies.

This book is not intended to replace the diagnosis, advice, or treatment healthcare professionals provide.

This book intends to pay homage to Barbara O'Neill's tireless work teaching people about herbal remedies while also seeking to guide others to live their lives holistically using the valuable information within.

Before using any herbal medicines in this book, seek a check-up with your healthcare professional to ensure that no remedy will cause unwarranted side effects or interact with any medications that may be taken.

Introduction

Herbal medicine has existed since ancient humans, predating any recorded history. It's believed that hunter-gatherers found plants, minerals, and even animal products that alleviated various ailments. Each tribe would teach the young, who would go on to teach their children as time passed. It's thanks to these early humans that we have the modern medicine that we use today. After all, if it weren't for the willow tree or the opium poppy, we wouldn't have aspirin or morphine.

However, this didn't happen overnight, as no one back then knew what it was within these herbal remedies that treated the ailments. Thankfully, as science matured, the active ingredients in the herbal remedies were identified and isolated. Once isolated, the active ingredients could be manufactured, and that was the birth of modern medicine.

Despite modern medicine being prescribed for everything from a rash to cancer, some still hold onto herbal remedies. Traditional medicines, such as Unani, traditional Chinese medicine, and Ayurveda, still use herbal remedies, but they aren't the only ones. Many people know that chamomile promotes sleep, while lavender eases stress and anxiety, and they use these remedies for those purposes despite the existence of pharmaceutical drugs that can achieve the same results. Why is that?

While many people require modern medicine, some are turning away from it for a variety of reasons:

- They fear pharmaceutical drugs and their possible side effects.

- They wish to break away from their dependency on pharmaceutical drugs.
- They prefer a more holistic approach to healing.
- They are tired of being prescribed standardized treatments that do nothing or worsen their symptoms.
- They want to be in control of their health.

There are even those who are losing faith in modern medicine. Modern medicine is often a reactive process, meaning that it treats the symptoms only after a person has gotten ill. While these symptoms should be treated, once they disappear, the medicine is stopped with no more questions asked. This results in underlying conditions remaining hidden and causing more problems later. The only time possible underlying conditions are explored is when the symptoms keep occurring even after several rounds of treatments.

While there is a place for reactive medicine, such as treating anaphylaxis or a broken bone, this reactive practice isn't always the best approach. Concentrating on symptoms or a specific body part can lead to missing important clues while treating a person.

Taking a proactive approach to medicine is considered more holistic. It helps prevent disease, lowers the risks of developing chronic conditions, and reduces existing symptoms. You can take a proactive approach to your health in many ways, such as reducing stress, improving sleep, improving diet, and being more active. Another proactive approach is to use herbal remedies to deal with problems before you approach your doctor.

You aren't required to always run to a doctor for every little sniffle. Echinacea is known to reduce the duration of colds and flu and ease their symptoms. Not only that, but it boosts the immune system, making your body hardier at fighting infections. Given that these are viral infections, medicine can't do much, and throat lozenges can only soothe the pain for so long.

Instead of treating the body like a jumble of parts that should be treated separately, it should be seen as a single entity with interconnected pieces. This approach extends beyond the physical body to include the mind and emotional well-being. If these two aren't in balance, the body will suffer. Treating it as a whole instead of its parts promotes overall strengthening and enhances the body's natural ability to heal itself.

I spent most of my life in Oregon, and while I had access to the hustle and bustle of city life, I felt the call of nature early on in life. Even today, I still prefer living closer to nature than I do living in the city, and it has made all the difference for me and my daughter. We have been living off the grid with our horse for seventeen years (as I write this page). And while this way of living offers many benefits, it hasn't been easy—especially in the beginning—as we were responsible for everything, including our health.

Rushing into town to see a doctor was a nightmare, but, in the beginning, I thought this was the only way. Thankfully, when you live off-grid, you quickly learn how to become self-sufficient, including looking after your health. I took my time learning about the different kinds of herbal medicines, particularly those I could make and use from the comfort of my own garden or foraging in the nearby woods.

While growing my herbal knowledge, I stumbled across the teachings of Barbara O'Neill, and I was *fascinated*. Unlike many other natural healers, she wasn't just preaching about living a healthy life aligned with nature—she also lived it herself, off the grid, just like me! So many of her teachings already aligned with how I was living my life, so with a few changes, it was easy to incorporate them into my existing lifestyle. Barbara suggested various herbal remedies that helped the body's natural ability to heal itself. It was so refreshing to see ways to build up the body's own immunity instead of just treating arising problems. Just like the title of the book suggests, she was a profound inspiration for writing this book.

Many years later, I am finally ready to share everything I have learned and developed through natural remedies to improve your life in ways you couldn't even imagine. I put together all my knowledge in this book on naturopathy to make your journey easier and healthier. I hope to inspire you to make small changes in your everyday life to enjoy a more holistic, self-sufficient lifestyle using what nature has always provided.

Within the pages of this book, you'll discover

- the guiding principles Barbara O'Neill lives by.
- the variety of herbal medicines and remedies for various ailments is safe for beginners and experienced users.
- all you need to make these remedies from the comfort of your own home.
- ways to help you reconnect the abundance and beauty of Mother Nature.
- tips on how to live well, and so much more.

With the ever-rising autoimmune diseases, cancer, obesity, insomnia, chronic inflammation, and mental health conditions, this book will be your handy guide to avoid the triggering additions that may already be part of your life.

This book provides a proactive approach to your health and integrates herbal remedies into your everyday life to improve your health and well-being. These remedies will help alleviate symptoms and even increase the chances of curing and preventing different health conditions.

Your body is your temple, and keeping it healthy will be strong enough to resist anything this modern day and age can throw at it. Each page is filled with treasured information, so don't stop here—turn the page to begin the first day of your new life.

Chapter 1: Getting to Know Barbara O'Neill and Her Philosophy

Barbara O'Neill has been instrumental in my decision to bring more herbal remedies into my life. Not only because of how they dealt with different ailments through the years but also because the goal of those remedies wasn't only to treat the ailments but to tackle the underlying problems that I didn't even know were brewing.

For those who are unfamiliar with Barbara O'Neill, she is originally from Australia and is a lover of nature. However, she is so much more. While trained in the ways of modern medicine, all her training came to naught when her firstborn daughter, Emma, became ill with an earache at 16 months old. After several rounds of antibiotics over six weeks, the earache kept recurring. As conventional medicine was unable to assist with the problems that stemmed from this diagnosis, Barbara embarked on a journey to find alternatives to help.

She went as far as spending 12 years in the New South Wales forest to develop the different philosophies she lives by today. While not heralded as a natural healer by all, Barbara has a large following of those who wish to improve their lives and well-being.

Barbara firmly believes that under the right conditions, our bodies are fully capable of healing themselves, which is true since a strong immune system can fight off a wide range of pathogenic microbes. Given her love of teaching others, Barbara has a large presence on YouTube, Facebook, and TikTok, allowing her to reach a wider audience. While she may not be everyone's cup of tea, I greatly respect what she does; her philosophies, principles, and teachings are invaluable in a world that should be looking toward proactive medicine instead of reactive medicine.

Getting to Know Barbara's Philosophies, Principles, and Teachings

As I learned more about Barbara, I took a lot of her teachings to heart and started living by them. While my own principles and philosophies have become entangled with hers, I would like to share some of my favorites that truly struck a chord.

Firstly, using herbal remedies is more than just prescribing herbs to fix a problem you may be having. It's about supporting a healthy healing process that involves various lifestyle changes to improve your life. Some of these changes can include lowering your exposure to pollution or irritants, improving your sleep hygiene, bettering your diet, getting more active, staying hydrated, supporting gut health, and reducing stress. In our modern society, it's all about getting things done now, resulting in late nights, poor diet, and surviving on caffeine. While occasional indulgences won't destroy your body, living this way constantly will cause a cascading effect of a variety of health conditions, especially chronic ones. You must be proactive to boost your health from the inside out.

It's necessary to maintain a healing environment. No matter how many lifestyle changes you make or herbal remedies you use, no changes will help for long if you continue to put yourself in unsupportive situations.

Your diet is an important factor when it comes to your body's condition. If you feed it poor-quality fuel, you won't get much quality function out of it. Small improvements—incorporating more whole foods (fruits and vegetables), whole grains, lean meat cuts, or plant-based proteins—are a great way to get started. These foods are known for their anti-inflammatory properties, which can help lower the risk of chronic conditions. Adding more fruits and vegetables, especially of different colors, is the best way to get phytonutrients (antioxidants in plants that protect the body), antioxidant compounds, and fiber. Remember, removing poor-quality or junk food from your diet will have a greater impact than just applying good habits. It's best to start by reducing and then stopping bad habits before starting good ones.

No one should be barred from receiving the medical care they need. Herbal remedies are affordable and can be grown, harvested, or purchased by anyone. When growing a medicinal garden or harvesting from nature, it's important to remember that nature should be respected. As long as you treat the plants out in nature with respect and give ample opportunity for harvested areas to regrow, nature will look after you with a healthy bounty.

Herbal remedies don't have to be complicated. A few peppermint leaves in a cup of hot water is enough to settle an upset stomach. However, for these remedies to be easy to put together, it's your responsibility to continue your education about the ingredients that go into each remedy. This book should guide you but shouldn't be your only resource. Continued education leads to more experience and confidence in what you're willing to try and test. Never allow your knowledge to stagnate, especially regarding potential risks, such as allergies and sensitivities. Chamomile is generally lauded as one of the best ways to fight insomnia. However, if you are allergic to ragweed or other daisy species, there is a strong chance you'll be allergic to chamomile.

Thankfully, lavender, passionflower, and valerian can also be used to fight insomnia. Be bold in your research.

Your body knows you better than you know it; learn to listen. Take your sleep cycle, for instance—it tells you that you're tired and need to rest. However, exposure to blue light from electronic devices can disrupt this cycle, keeping you awake longer than is healthy and causing difficulty in falling asleep. Insufficient healthy sleep can lead to problems such as insomnia, anxiety, and other issues. Yet the sleep cycle isn't the only cycle by which we can be influenced. Consider the seasons and what nature provides during them. It's no coincidence that citrus fruits, lauded for having high vitamin C, are readily available during the colder months when colds and flu are more common. Vitamin C is an antioxidant that helps bolster the immune system to fight pathogenic microorganisms, including viruses that cause flu and colds. Eating seasonally isn't only beneficial for your health but also your budget, as eating readily available foods is cheaper than eating those grown out of season.

Taking care of your mental and emotional health is crucial in today's times. One of the best ways to do that is through self-care. Self-care varies from person to person, so don't expect what works for someone on Instagram to work for you. Some people feel at home in a forest, while others prefer hitting the gym or bathing with a good book. As long as you're taking the time to look after your health—body, mind, and spirit—then that is self-care. However, keep in mind that not everything you may do to relax is considered good for your body, so be sure to check that you're helping yourself and not hindering your health.

While Barbara's many other teachings may impact your life, these are the ones that most spoke to me. I encourage you to go forth and find out more about her and what she has to offer the world and you.

Chapter 2: Understanding Herbal Medicine and Remedies

The origins of herbal remedies are shrouded in mystery, but there are clues to their usage in early humans. In 1960, a groundbreaking discovery was made in the Shanidar Cave, Iraq: the body of a Neanderthal found buried with several known medicinal plants. The body is believed to be 60,000–80,000 years old, which suggests that even our prehistoric ancestors were already tapping into nature's medicinal properties.

Cave paintings found in Lascaux Caves, France, noted more evidence of the use of herbal remedies. These paintings not only depict some plants believed to have medicinal properties but also date back to 25,000–13,000 B.C.E.

Another body, that of a modern man named Ötzi, also known as Iceman, was discovered in 1991 in the Swiss Alps. He was found with birch fungus (*Piptoporus betulinus*). This fungus was believed to have been used as a way to deal with internal parasites due to its antibacterial and antibiotic properties. The body was determined to be over 5,300 years old.

The first written account of an herbal remedy was the use of willow bark documented on a stone tablet dating back to the Third Dynasty of Ur, roughly 3000 B.C.E. From there, as the written and spoken word traveled across the world, more remedies were being documented and used by those who had access to the plants involved.

Science was in its infancy, but as it developed, those who practiced it wanted to know what was in the herbal remedies that made them so effective. Once science was advanced enough, active ingredients were identified as the compounds that were healing the conditions.

Once the active ingredients were identified, they could be isolated and produced on a larger scale. Bringing medicine to people worldwide, bringing about the birth of pharmaceutical drugs.

However, unlike herbal remedies, these drugs underwent stringent clinical testing, allowing them to be safe for most people while identifying possible side effects. Despite the access to modern medicine, many still turn to herbal medicine. These remedies are often more cost-effective and accessible, as there is no need for a prescription; they have a natural origin with minimal side effects and empower people to take their health into their own hands.

However, it's important to realize that herbal medicines aren't intended to replace but complement modern medicine. They, too, have their side effects and contraindications, and this is why it's so important to discuss herbal medicine usage with your doctor to prevent possible herb-drug interactions. Even if there isn't a known interaction, people are unique, and there is a chance that an herbal remedy may affect them differently than others. Hence, why it's so necessary to listen to what your body is telling you.

When you think of an herb, you may only consider the leaves of a particular plant, but herbal remedies are more than that. All parts of a plant can be used to make herbal remedies, including roots, berries, flowers, bark, and more. In some cases, multiple parts of the same plant can be used to treat different ailments. For instance, dandelion leaves are known to be a diuretic, allowing the body to flush excess fluid, which, in turn, can assist in flushing the kidneys and bladder of potential pathogens. However, the root is often used to stimulate appetite as well as bolster the health of the gallbladder and liver. It can also be roasted and ground into a coffee substitute.

While single-herb remedies are common, combinations or blends of herbs can often be more effective than individual herbs alone. This is due to the synergy that herbs can have with one another. Unlike pharmaceutical drugs, which typically have an additive effect, herbal blends can have a multiplicative effect, helping the body maintain a healthy balance without the risk of a potential overdose.

This potency is attributed to the various compounds found in herbs, such as polyphenols, which help to protect the body. In contrast, pharmaceutical drugs contain high concentrations of active ingredients and none of the protective compounds.

A well-known example of this synergy is turmeric and black pepper. Turmeric is known for its anti-inflammatory properties, which are due to its active ingredient, curcumin. Unfortunately, curcumin isn't bioavailable upon digestion. However, when consumed with piperine, the active ingredient in black pepper, curcumin's bioavailability increases, allowing more of it to be absorbed.

However, synergy will only go so far, and in order to make personal blends, the necessary knowledge needs to be gained through research and subsequent experimentation. You must understand what benefits certain plants can offer, as well as the dangers they can pose.

It's not only how herbal remedies work that you need to understand, but also what other foods and drinks you consume can affect the absorption. For instance, while coffee may help wake you up in the morning, it can also interfere with the absorption of certain supplements. To mitigate this, the consumption of coffee and supplements should happen at different times of the day. Your overall diet will also influence how well herbal remedies work for you. Taking an herbal remedy to combat inflammation may be ineffective if you continue to consume foods and drinks that promote inflammation.

You don't even need to create an herbal remedy to benefit from it. Many herbs can be eaten as is, added to foods, or blended into sauces or drinks. As long as you understand the herbs you're adding to your diet, the addition will help improve your health and well-being.

Now that you have a better understanding of herbal remedies and medicine, it's time to see what you'll need to make your own herbal blends and preparations.

Chapter 3: Requirements to Make Herbal Remedies

To make a cake, you need both specific ingredients and tools to make it as perfect as possible. Similarly, crafting various herbal remedies requires having the right tools and quality ingredients to ensure their effectiveness.

Tools

Tools can be divided into preparation and harvesting. Whether harvesting from a garden or foraging, it's important to use sharp and clean tools. Keep shears, scissors, knives, trowels, and a hand lens handy. Not only will these tools help you collect what you need, but you'll also be able to identify what you're collecting—especially when foraging.

Foraging can be a rewarding practice, but it can also be dangerous if you're not well-informed about the plants that grow in your area. That's why it's crucial to educate yourself. Investing in field guides and taking opportunities to go on guided foraging tours are excellent ways to learn what is safe to collect. Other books you may want to invest in include other herbal remedy books or medicinal herb books. Keeping a notebook or two will also be handy in the long run.

The tools you'll need will depend on the types of preparations you want to make. Infusions don't require many tools, but making salves will require more. Some of the best tools you should have can be found in the list below:

- Different kinds of kitchen tools assist with measuring and mixing. It's also a good idea to have a kettle so that hot water is always on hand. A grater will be required when using wax blocks. Different-sized funnels will help with decanting liquid into different-sized containers.

  If you'd like to make capsules, you'll need to grind herbs and spices finely. You can use a mortar and pestle or a coffee grinder.

- Straining tools will help to remove solids from liquids, so include cheesecloths, mesh strainers, tea balls, and even Fresh presses in your arsenal. While the latter two can be used for smaller volumes, the aforementioned are best for larger volumes.

- You'll need many different types of containers, depending on what preparation you're making. When using vinegar or alcohol, always use glass. For everything else, use BPA-food-grade plastics, as this won't contaminate or compromise your herbal remedies. Some of the best containers are tins (salves), jars (tea blends), and amber-colored bottles (alcohol extractions).

- When using butter and waxes, you'll need a double boiler. This will also assist in making heated oil infusions and prevent burning your remedies.

- Labels are vital for identifying what is in the containers in which you store your remedies. You will never have enough labels.

Ideally, you should look at the recipes you'd like to try and determine the required tools.

Ingredients

Botanicals (all plant material) are one of the main ingredients you'll be using to make herbal medicine. While it's possible to forage and grow enough to suit your needs, if you want to make larger quantities of preparations you'd like to share, or if any of these herbal remedies aren't locally available, you may find yourself in a situation where you'd have to purchase botanical ingredients.

When doing this, it's important to use companies that harvest or source ethically, share the same values you do, and have the necessary certifications, particularly if you want organic botanicals. If you have an apothecary or herbalist in your area, you can make your purchases through them.

However, this isn't always possible, but thankfully, some companies are known for their quality and ethically harvested herbs. For those living in North America, Mountain Rose Herbs and Frontier Co-op are great options. If you need shipping internationally, look no further than Bulk Apothecary and Pacific Botanicals.

While botanicals will make up the bulk of your creations, they are by no means the only additions to your ingredient list. Before you get excited and buy everything that looks interesting, it's a good idea to review your recipes to determine what you need, so nothing goes to waste. Consider these other ingredients:

- Solvents to use in your extractions and infusions. Those you will likely purchase are oils (including carrier oils), different kinds of vinegar, alcohol (good quality), and honey.

    - In most cases, quality vodka is good enough for a tincture, but unflavored gin and brandy will also do. Check the proof of the recipe before purchasing the alcohol.

- Waxes and butters are used with many skin preparations, such as salves and creams. Beeswax is most frequently used, but for vegan-friendly options, you can also consider soy, carnauba, and candelilla. Butters you can consider are various and include kokum, almond, avocado, and cocoa, to name a few.

    - Due to their strength, essential oils need to be diluted with a carrier oil to prevent damage to the skin. Some of the best include apricot kernel oil, sweet almond oil, olive oil, coconut oil, castor oil, and grapeseed oil. It's possible to be allergic to these oils, so a patch test will be required.

- Essential oils are powerful plant extracts often used in aromatherapy and various skin preparations. When purchasing them, it's important to note the cost, the color of the bottle (should be dark), whether the Latin name of the plant is present, the purity of the oil (should be 100%), and whether it has a source or certification.

Some of these ingredients can be pricey, especially the different kinds of oils and essential oils. Research what alternatives can be used if you find your budget can't handle a particular recipe.

Importance of Note-Keeping

If it's not documented, it didn't happen. There is nothing worse than failing to take notes when developing a new herbal remedy and forgetting how you made it. Having a notebook will allow you to keep track of your creations and how they affect you. It's also a great place to keep recipes you're testing, as well as information about your garden or great foraging spots.

While you should be labeling your creations, it's also a good idea to keep track of what you have in your notebook, so be sure to write preparations and dosages in there for quick referencing. It's also a great place to make notes of possible contraindications the preparations can cause.

Having quality tools and ingredients is a must if you want to make quality preparations. Now that you know what tools and ingredients you need, it's time to get familiar with the different kinds of preparations.

If you're enjoying this book, I'd be incredibly grateful if you could take a moment to leave a review or rating on the platform where you got it. Believe it or not, less than 1% of readers take the time to do so—your support would mean so much. Thank you!

Chapter 4: Exploring Different Preparations

Many different preparations target different parts of the body, using a variety of botanicals. Some of these preparations are easy enough for beginners, while others are more advanced. Take your time getting familiar with the different preparations, as this will assist you with the later herbal remedy chapters. Experiment with different preparations to get more comfortable with the techniques.

Infusions

An infusion is a type of extraction but is considered the weakest of the extractions, typically using solvents such as water or oil. The most well-known infusion is tea. Water infusions are normally done with hot or just boiled water, and the steeping time can be between 10–15 minutes, depending on what botanical is being used. Water infusions are most commonly ingested, while oil infusions tend to be reserved for skin preparations. You can use culinary herbs infused with edible oils, such as olive oil as well.

Oil infusions have the medicinal properties of botanicals absorbed into them over several weeks or longer, recipe-dependent. They have a longer shelf life, especially when made with dried herbs and the addition of vitamin E oil. An oil infusion made with fresh herbs can last up to three months in the fridge, but when made with dried herbs, it can last as long as a year when stored in a cool, dry area.

When these oils are stored at room temperature or exposed to fluctuating temperatures, they can go rancid in as few as 10 days. Water infusions don't last long—usually a few days—and need to be stored in the fridge.

Water Infusion Instructions

When you decide to make a water infusion, consider whether you want to make a blend or a single herb preparation. When making a blend, consider the ratios of the ingredients to make as much as you need. A dried blend can be stored for later use. This isn't possible with fresh herbs, as they need to be used as soon as they're picked.

- Boil the water.
- Add 2–3 teaspoons of the dried blend or single herb. When using fresh botanicals, you will need 2–3 tablespoons.
    - If you enjoy a stronger infusion, take 1–2 tablespoons of dried herbs or 3–5 tablespoons of fresh herbs.
- Allow the mixture to steep for up to 15 minutes, longer if using dried roots, dried berries, or bark.
- Strain the mixture, and squeeze any excess moisture out.
- Optionally, you can add a natural sweetener, such as honey maple syrup.

Dried herbs can last up to a year when stored in a sealed container placed in a cool, dry area. Any botanical considered edible can be used in a water infusion. Experiment with single herbs or herbal blends.

Water infusions are perfect for the more delicate botanicals, such as leaves and flowers. If herbs tend to be a little bitter, avoid steeping them longer than five minutes, as it may make the infusion too bitter to enjoy. This includes herbs such as citrus peels, lavender, and chamomile. Lightly crushing fresh herbs will allow more of their essential oils to be released in the hot water.

Oil Infusion Instructions

Oil infusions can be done with fresh or dried herbs. However, when making an infusion with fresh herbs, you'll need more volume than with dried herbs. The moisture content of the herbs will also impact the shelf life of the oil. So, if you aim to use fresh herbs, allow them to wilt for up to 12 hours before starting the infusion process. It's also a good idea to cut them into smaller pieces or even grind them slightly with the pestle and mortar. The quantity of herbs you will need will depend on the container you are using.

Folk Method

The folk method is the slow method and is great if you're not in a rush to get your infused oil.

- If using fresh herbs, fill the glass container, leaving only 1–2 inches headspace. If using dried herbs, only fill the container a third, as they will swell over time.
- Cover the herbs with at least an inch of oil of choice.

- Stir the mixture and top up the oil as needed.
- Seal the container and place it in a sunny, warm area. Shake the container daily.
- While the fresh herbs shouldn't need extra oil, the dried herbs will. So, top up as needed to keep them below the oil. Any herbs exposed to the air may become moldy.
- After the oil infuses for about 4 weeks, use cheesecloth to strain solids.
- Decant the infused oil into a clean bottle, seal it, and add a label. Store the container appropriately.
- Add vitamin E oil to the mixture to improve shelf life. It should make up 1% of the old solution.

It's not always possible to keep all the herbs below the oil level. If this occurs and mold starts to develop, scoop it out as soon as you notice it.

Heat Method

If you want access to your infused oil within a few days, the heat method is for you.

- Fresh and dried can be used, but remember that fresh herbs will impact the shelf life of the oil.
- Add the herbs you wish to use to a double boiler and add enough oil to cover them by 1–2 inches.
- Bring the temperature of the stove to 100–140 °F and allow the oil to heat for 1–5 hours. Consider the oil ready when it takes on the scent and color of the herbs you're using.

    - If keeping the oil at 100 °F, the infusion can take as long as 48–72 hours, depending on the botanical you're using.

- Allow to fully cool.
- Pour the oil through a cheesecloth to strain out any solids and squeeze excess oil out of the solids.
- Transfer the oil to a sealable container, seal it, label it, and store it appropriately.
- As with the folk method, vitamin E oil can improve shelf life.

While many herbs can be used to make infused oils, some of the best include arnica, calendula, hot peppers (cayenne), mullein, rosemary, and thyme.

Decoctions

Decoctions are similar to infusions, but instead of the botanicals steeping in hot water, they're gently simmered in water to extract more compounds. Decoctions are the perfect preparation for tough botanicals such as barks, berries, and roots, regardless of whether they are fresh or dried. Decoctions can be too bitter if the simmering time isn't observed in some recipes.

Some of the best botanicals to use for decoctions are roots (astragalus and burdock), berries (hawthorn and goji), citrus peels, seeds (fenugreek and coriander), and barks (wild cherry and cinnamon). If using fresh ingredients, ensure that they are thoroughly washed before chopping them into pieces and making a decoction. Dried botanicals should also be chopped into smaller pieces before getting started. The larger surface area allows for more beneficial compounds to be pulled from the botanicals. If the decoctions are in a sealed container in the fridge, they can last up to 72 hours.

Decoction Instructions

Decoctions allow for more mineral salts and various bitter compounds to be extracted.

1. In a saucepan, add a pint of water to an ounce of cut or macerated dried botanicals before bringing the mixture to a gentle simmer.

2. Allow the mixture to simmer without the lid until the volume is reduced by a quarter. The liquid should change color to be similar to the herbs used.

3. Remove from the heat. If also using delicate leaves or flowers in the recipe, add them to the mixture and add a lid, allowing the botanicals to steep for a further 10–15 minutes.

4. After steeping the delicate botanicals, strain the solids out of the mixture.

5. The decoction can be enjoyed hot or cooled completely before storing.

6. Retain the liquid in a clean container, seal it, label it, and store it in the fridge to use as needed.

For a smaller recipe, you can use 3 tablespoons of dried botanicals to a quart of water.

Extracts

Infusions and decoctions are a type of extraction that extracts the water- and oil-soluble compounds in the botanicals using water as a solvent. Botanicals have many different compounds or constituents within them, and they can be extracted using a range of solvents. The different solvents give rise to various types of extractions, as they make for powerful herbal remedies. The kinds of extract made with different solvents include:

- Oil infusions allow for the extraction of essential oils and other fat-soluble compounds. This method is suited to calendula and comfrey.
- Honey infusions are a great way to combine the benefits of honey with the benefits of the herbs infused in it. A honey infusion can last about six months.
- Hydrosols is a type of extraction using water to extract water-soluble compounds. This method is often used to make rose water or witch hazel extract. This method is ideal for rose, willow, and witch hazel.
- Acetum is a vinegar extraction that extracts minerals, vitamins, and trace elements. Botanicals such as parsley and stinging nettle work well in acetum. While white spirit vinegar is usually used, many people opt to use apple cider vinegar due to the additional benefits this vinegar offers.

- Alcohol extracts, such as tinctures, are considered among the strongest available. They can be applied to most botanicals but are ideal for tougher varieties. Tinctures can last up to 10 years but will start losing potency after this time. All alcohol extracts need to be stored in small, dark bottles to prevent evaporation.

- Glycerites are glycerin extracts that are only second to alcohol extracts in terms of herbal remedy strength. Unlike alcohol, glycerin can extract saponins, a compound that helps bolster the immune system to fight cancer and assists in reducing cholesterol levels. This type of extract has a shelf life of 14–24 months.

Extracts can be stored longer than other herbal remedies, and because of this, there may be a few physical changes. If plants with resins have been used, there is a chance that the resin will precipitate and create crystals, and the liquid may separate into layers. The extract can still be used if this occurs. While alcohol extracts won't develop mold, the others may, and once this occurs, the extract should be thrown away.

Oxymel Instructions

Oxymels, a type of extract, are a unique extraction where honey and vinegar are used to extract a range of compounds from the botanicals used. The most well-known oxymel is fire cider, which is often used to support the immune system as the weather starts to cool. While there are many ways to make an oxymel, the following is the easiest method but is by no means the only method. Most botanicals can be used with this method, although it's better to use dried herbs.

1. In a pint jar, add enough dried herbs to fill a quarter of the volume.

2. Pour in equal parts vinegar of choice and honey, keeping 1–2 inches headspace.

3. Stir well with a wooden skewer to ensure the herbs are well coated and the honey is dissolved in the vinegar.

4. Clean the jar's rims before adding the lid. Ideally, a plastic lid should be used as the acidity can cause the lid to rust. Alternatively, a piece of parchment paper can be placed between the jar and the rim to prevent the mixture from touching the lid directly.

5. Give the jar a good shake, as this helps to macerate the contents and help with the release of beneficial compounds.

6. Place in a cool, dark area for at least 2 weeks. Shake at least twice a week.

7. After the extraction process is complete, strain the solids from the oxymel, squeezing to get all the liquid available.

8. Decant the oxymel into a fresh container and seal it with the appropriate lid. Label appropriately and store in a cool, dark area.

Oxymels generally have a shelf life of six months. Great herbs to use in an oxymel include but aren't limited to, rosemary, lemon peel, garlic, lemon balm, elderberries, and dandelions. Any honey can be used to make an oxymel. If you want to add unique tastes to your oxymel, look into using different floral honeys.

Oxymels are usually safe for all to enjoy; however, because honey is used, it shouldn't be given to children under the age of one.

Tincture Instructions

Tinctures—especially those made with alcohol—can be potent and are generally used to extract compounds that can't be extracted with water, such as resins and alkaloids. Tinctures can be made with fresh or dried herbs. When using fresh herbs, add enough to fill a jar, but if using dry, only use enough to fill a quarter of the container's volume.

1. Use preferred herbs, either dry or fresh. Fresh herbs can be packed into the jar.

2. Fill the jar with the preferred alcohol, vinegar, or glycerin, depending on the type of extraction you want to achieve.

3. Seal the container—adding parchment paper if using vinegar—then label and store in a cool, dark area for the next six weeks.

4. Shake the contents at least once a day.

5. After extraction, strain the liquid from the solids, squeezing any excess from the solids.

6. Pour the retained liquid into a clean container before sealing it, labeling it, and storing it in a cool, dry area until required.

7. The shelf-life of the tincture will be dependent on what solvent is used. The type of solvent used with determine the shelf-life of the tincture.

The best fresh herbs to use for tinctures include valerian, echinacea, and lemon balm, while for dry herbs, try using cardamon, lavender, or astragalus.

When using alcohol, you can use grain alcohols, vodka, gin, and whiskey, as long as there are no artificial additives or flavors. Pay careful concentration to the alcohol proof you use, as certain proofs are better from fresh, dried, or resin-rich botanicals.

Botanicals with resin or fresh plant materials do well with 190-proof alcohol (95%). This is also true for 151-proof alcohol (75%). Alcohols that are 100-proof (50%) are perfect for fresh or dried, though the fresh material should be slightly wilted. The 80-proof alcohol (40%) can be used for fresh herbs but is best suited for dry botanical material.

Poultices

A poultice is a mixture of botanicals or minerals combined with a liquid to make a paste that can be applied to the skin. Also known as a cataplasm, the mixture has long been used to promote healing and lowering inflammation in rashes, insect bites, or stings and drawing out infection from wounds, cysts, and abscesses.

Various ingredients can be used to make a poultice. While there are botanicals such as turmeric, garlic, mullein, aloe, and dandelion that can be used, there are various others that are just as effective. Some people swear by bread and milk, clay, grated raw potatoes, and even baking soda. The liquids used to make the paste are also variable, including water, honey, milk, or preferred oil. The reason for the various ingredients is due to the application to the skin and the chance of different allergies and sensitivities occurring.

Poultices can also be heated to help draw out infection more effectively. However, if using this method, ensure the poultice is warm but never hot, to prevent the skin from being burnt. Never apply a poultice to an open wound, as this can irritate the healing wound or worsen the infection. Add the poultice to some cheesecloth and create a compress that can be added to the injury.

Poultice Instructions

The herbs you use in a poultice will depend on what you're trying to heal. Basil leaves are great for bug bites, while bread and milk can help remove a splinter, and chamomile can assist in drawing out an infection in an abscess. Research the effects of different herbs to determine which is best to use. Regardless of which botanical you decide to use, ensure that it is edible to prevent poisoning yourself. Poultices are best made from fresh botanicals.

1. Select the fresh herbs of your choice and wash thoroughly before patting dry. If the herbs selected have stalks or branches, remove these and only use the leaves.

2. The amount of botanical you'll need will depend on the affected area. There is no right or wrong measurement.

3. Add the botanicals to a mortar and 1–2 teaspoons of the preferred liquid. Use the pestle to crush the mixture into a uniform paste. Add more liquid or botanicals to get the thickness you prefer. Grind the mixture for 1–2 minutes.

4. If you don't have a pestle and mortar, you can mash the mixture in a bowl, making it as uniform as possible.

5. Before adding the poultice to the affected area, wash it thoroughly with soap and water. Take the time to wash your hands as well.

6. Apply the poultice to the affected area with a spoon and spread it thinly with your fingers.

7. If applying to a large area, add some gauze and a bandage to keep the poultice in place. A bandage can cover a smaller area, size dependent on the injury.

8. Check the poultice every 4–6 hours to ensure that if there is an infection, it is under control and not spreading. It's important to monitor wounds so you can act accordingly.

9. A fresh poultice should be made and applied to the injury.

A poultice doesn't even need to be overly complicated. Chewing plantain (the weed) leaves and then applying it straight to a bug bite or even a zit will help reduce the inflammation and itchiness, and assist in healing.

Inhalations

Inhalations combine the essential oils in botanicals with steam, making an effective remedy to deal with respiratory problems. Using inhalations can assist with opening sinuses, moistening the mucus membranes in the nasal passages, and even loosening mucus buildup in the chest and sinuses.

Many herbs can be used in inhalation blends, from mild herbs such as lavender, mullein, basil, and mint to stronger botanicals such as eucalyptus and tea tree oil. You don't even need to use botanicals if you can't find them dried or fresh. Essential oils hold many benefits from their botanicals, and they are powerful extracts. All you need are a few drops to get a powerful inhalation.

Inhalation Instructions

There are various ways to inhale herbal remedies. The following instructions are for an inhalation method that is most frequently used by those who want to clear their sinuses due to colds or hay fever. For the best results, use dried herbs. If using fresh herbs, use 3 times the amount as described for dry herbs.

1. Boil 2 quarts of water and add it to a heatproof bowl.
2. Add up to 2 hands full of herbs to the water and allow it to steep for 10 minutes.
3. You can add a few drops of your preferred essential oil into the water.
4. Drape a large towel over your head so it covers the bowl and creates a tent, trapping the steam in it.
5. Inhale the stream while your eyes are closed. Breathe in through your nose and out through your mouth for 10 breaths. Then switch and breathe through your mouth and out your nose for the next 10 breaths. Continue for up to 10 minutes.

6. If the heat is too much, or the scent burns your nose, take a break and try again until the clogged sinuses open.

While effective, be careful—the steam can burn your skin, and the oils can burn your eyes while open. Frequent treatments of this inhalation method can irritate the skin, so don't make the sessions longer than 15 minutes, and don't repeat more than 3 times a day.

If you're concerned about being too close to the steam and essential oils, add the herbs to your bath water or tie a scent bag to the shower head. This will create a sauna effect in the bathroom with the necessary botanicals to help open your sinuses.

An alternative inhalation method is aromatherapy. Aromatherapy can be as simple as sniffing the contents of an essential oil bottle or more complicated as using a diffuser. However, if using a diffuser, ensure that they're used in open rooms and away from children and pets, as consuming essential oils is dangerous.

Skin Treatments

When it comes to skin treatments, many different preparations range from infused oils to a variety of types of creams, ointments, balms, and salves. The preparation you decide to use is dependent on the task that needs to be completed. Which you decide to use depends on what formulation you prefer over others and what the intent of the preparation is. The only real difference between the different formulations is the ratios between the wax, infused oils, and butter. Most homemade skin treatments will last 6–12 months.

Ointments

Ointments are the softest of the preparations. Ointments are usually used to treat problems, such as rashes, eczema, irritation, and itchiness. Ointments are highly absorbent as they are oil-based formulations. The semi-solid viscosity is easily absorbed but tends to leave a greasy residue until it's fully absorbed. The oil content of ointments tends to be as high as 80%, while the remaining portion is either wax or a type of butter.

Ointment Instructions

Due to the softness of ointments, they are gentle enough to be used on most parts of the body, even the face. While there are many different recipes for ointments, it's a good idea to carefully look at the ratio between wax and oil to see how soft the ointment will be.

1. Take 1.7–3.5 ounces of dried herbs or 3.5–7 ounces of fresh herbs, and place them in a saucepan with 27 ounces of your preferred oil (olive, coconut, jojoba, and so on).

2. Raise the temperature to 100–140°F and stir, allowing the oil to slowly heat. Once the oil takes on the color of the herb and the oil is steaming, then remove it from the heat.

3. Allow the oil to cool enough to handle and strain the solids out.

4. Return the infused oil and 5.3 ounces of beeswax to a double boiler. Raise the temperature to medium and slowly melt the wax, stirring with a wooden skewer. Remove from heat once melted.

5. Cool the mixture for 1-2 minutes and then add 20-100 drops of your favorite essential oil. Add 8 ounces of herb-infused oil and an ounce of beeswax to a double boiler

6. Transfer the ointment to prepared tins and allow them to cool to room temperature before sealing them, labeling them, and storing them in a cool, dark place. Ointments can last up to 6 months.

Salves

Salves are harder than ointments as they contain more wax. These skin preparations are usually used to soothe the sore muscles and treat inflammation and other ailments. Due to their thickness, they aren't as absorbent as ointments but create a layer on the skin that protects it.

Salve Instructions

Have an herbal-infused oil ready to save time when preparing a salve. Refer to the oil infusion instructions to make one.

1. Add 8 ounces of herb-infused oil and an ounce of beeswax to a double boiler. Heat over medium until the wax is fully melted.

2. Check the consistency by dipping a spoon in the mixture and placing it in the freezer for a few minutes. Rub the salve between your fingers to determine its thickness. Thicken the mixture by adding more wax.

3. Once its reached the desired consistency, allow the mixture to cool and add any essential oils you may want.

4. Pour the salve into the waiting containers and allow to cool to room temperature.
5. Seal, label, and store the container in a cool, dark area. It can last up to a year.

Balms

Balms are the most solid of the skin preparations and tend to retain their shape (think of lip balm) unless temperatures are high.

It also has the highest wax content of the skin preparations. It's easy to turn a salve into a balm by reducing the infused oil volume.

1. Add 6 ounces of infused oil and an ounce of beeswax to a double boiler.
2. Raise the temperature to medium until the wax is melted and incorporated into the oil.
3. Test the consistency and adjust oil or wax as needed to get the thickness required.
4. Cool for a few minutes before adding any essential oils.
5. Pour into clean containers and allow to fully cool before sealing it.
6. Label containers before storing them in a cool, dark area. Balms will last roughly a year when stored correctly.

Diluting Essential Oils

There will be times that you don't want to make an infused oil but rather want to use essential oils to get the same effect. This is possible, but it's important to remember that essential oils cannot be used directly on the skin due to their strength. If you're going to add essential oils to your skin, you need to dilute them first.

In most cases, a 3% dilution is perfect for any skin preparation. This can be achieved by adding 1/4 teaspoon of essential oil to an ounce of carrier oil (Gomez, 2022).

However, if applying essential oils to children, the dilution should be as low as 1%, or 6 drops of essential oil to an ounce of carrier oil. If you want to make a blend of essential oils, it's best to mix the blend of essential oils, place it in a container with a dropper, and mix well before diluting.

These are only some of the available preparations you can use in your herbal remedy journey. It's encouraged for you to discover others you may want to use as you expand your research. Now that you have an understanding of some of the most common preparations, it's time to explore the safety concerns and contraindications surrounding herbal remedies and how you can protect yourself.

Chapter 5: Safety and Contraindications

Unlike pharmaceutical drugs, which undergo stringent clinical testing, herbal remedies aren't as thoroughly tested. The Food and Drug Administration (FDA) doesn't regulate herbal remedies and considers them dietary supplements, despite the considerable anecdotal evidence that shows how their use can improve well-being.

Despite not being considered medicine, herbal remedies have something in common with pharmaceutical drugs: they can cause side effects and interact with other herbs and medications.

Ideally, herbal medicine aims not to harm those who use it, but due to the active ingredients and other compounds within the botanicals, along with the uniqueness of individuals, there is always a chance that a negative outcome can be experienced.

For this reason, before using any herbal remedy, even one you make, discuss it with your medical practitioner, experienced naturopath, or other herbalist.

These professionals can inform you about possible interactions and monitor the effects of the remedy, whether it's positive or not.

However, they shouldn't be your only source of information. Continue your research and stay aware of potential interactions that could cause problems. Keep educating yourself and always use quality ingredients.

Side Effects

Because of the various compounds found within botanicals, there is always a chance of side effects. Some can be mild, such as headaches, digestive issues, and nausea, while others can be more severe, such as allergic reactions, heart palpitations, increased blood pressure, or hormones being affected. This is why it is crucial to speak with your healthcare provider, especially when it comes to dosage. Something as simple as licorice can have devastating effects if the dosage is incorrect.

Licorice contains glycyrrhizin and, in high concentrations, can cause pseudoaldosteronism, a hormonal disorder that can increase blood pressure and even result in a heart attack. Even foods considered good for you can be deadly when the dosage is incorrect. Dark green leafy vegetables are known for their health benefits; however, they contain oxalates, and if eaten in high concentrations, they can increase the chance of kidney stones, which can damage the kidneys. These are only some of the side effects that can occur; there are many others, more so if allergies, intolerances, and sensitivities come into play.

Patch Test

While it's not a good idea to consume something you may be allergic to, you can do the patch test to determine if you're allergic to a specific topical application to test for a possible allergen. Some preparations include teas (used as washes), all types of creams, carrier oils, poultices, and infused oils.

1. Ideally, the patch test should be done on a small piece of sensitive skin, such as the inside of the wrist or elbow crook. Thoroughly wash the area with soap and water before patting dry.

2. Add the preparation you're testing to the cleaned area and cover with some gauze and a bandage or Band-Aid.

3. Leave the patch to remain in place for at least 24 hours.

4. After the test is complete, remove the patch and scrutinize your skin. If you note swelling, hives, redness, itchiness, or any pain, it's best to avoid that particular remedy.

5. If you note any of these adverse reactions before the 24 hours have passed, immediately remove the patch and wash the area. If symptoms worsen, seek medical attention.

When doing a patch test, avoid using any blends, as this will make it more difficult to determine which botanical or oil may be causing the problem.

Understanding Interactions

Just as there are drug-drug interactions that prevent certain medications from being taken together, there are also herb-drug interactions. These interactions can enhance or reduce the effectiveness of other herbal remedies or medicines you're taking, which can have serious consequences.

Something as simple as garlic can thin the blood, and when taken with warfarin (a blood thinner), it can increase the chance of bleeding and bruising. Not only that but the effectiveness of saquinavir—a drug used to treat HIV—can be reduced by garlic.

St. John's wort is often used as an herbal remedy to help enhance mood, assisting with fighting anxiety and depression. However, it can affect the effectiveness of oral contraception and a range of other medications. Even goldenseal, often used to settle digestive issues, has a high herb-drug interaction with many kinds of medicines.

If you're curious about the possible herb-drug interactions, WebMD has a drug interaction checker you can use. However, it's always better to discuss the use of herbs and pharmaceutical drugs with your doctor to be safe.

You'll also need to consider the duration that an herbal remedy is taken for. While some can be used for the long term, not all of them can. For instance, echinacea, often used to treat colds and flu, shouldn't be taken longer than eight weeks.

While it's possible and safe to combine herbal remedies with modern medicine, it must be done safely, and under the guidance of medical professionals. However, not all herbal remedies are safe for everyone. As with most medications, not all herbal remedies are likely safe to use for those who are pregnant, breastfeeding, the very young, the very old, those who may be on specific medication, or those suffering certain conditions. Even caution needs to be taken when drinking herbal teas.

Now that you know how to keep yourself safe and have consulted with your healthcare provider about using alternative medicine, it's time to put your knowledge to the test. It's time to start making your own home remedies.

Chapter 6: First Aid Remedies

It's always a good idea to deal with minor emergencies yourself instead of clogging up a doctor's office or the emergency room. I had to learn this quickly while living off the grid, miles away from the nearest town.

Giving yourself and your loved ones the necessary first aid when needed is a vital skill, especially if some common ailments and injuries keep occurring. There are many different herbal remedies you can use to treat first-aid-worthy ailments, such as insect bites or controlling bruising.

It would also be beneficial to get the necessary first aid courses—all three if possible—as this will give you the training to recognize when a situation is out of your depth and requires professional help.

Insect Bites and Stings

Ranging from insects to arachnids, there are many creepy crawlies that bite. Some may pose problems if they are venomous or if there is an allergic reaction to the bite.

Generally, all you'll be left with is a red, itchy, and irritated welt. The itching can drive people to damage their skin and introduce bacteria that can cause infections.

Thankfully, there are many different ways that you can deal with the problem.

Remedies

The following remedies are mixtures of herbal and folk remedies that are used to treat the pain, inflammation, and itchiness associated with bug bites and stings.

- **Ice** can be added to a cloth before being placed on a bug bite for 10–15 minutes.

- **Oatmeal** can be used as a poultice or a bath to soothe the irritation. To make a poultice, mix equal parts oatmeal and water to make a thick paste and apply it to the skin. Leave it in place for 10 minutes before washing it away. For the bath, take a cup of oatmeal and allow it to steep in a bathtub with hot water. Once the water is tepid, lie in the tub for up to 20 minutes. This remedy also helps with sunburn.

- A **baking soda** poultice requires a tablespoon of baking soda with a few drops of water, just enough to make a paste. Apply the poultice to the affected area and leave it in place for 10 minutes. You can also crush up **aspirin** tablets to create a similar paste.

- A slice of fresh **onion** can be applied to the skin to reduce the inflammation of the injury.

- A dab of **toothpaste** will help alleviate itching.

- **Aloe vera** is often used to soothe all forms of skin irritation. Cut a leaf open and scrape the clear gel out, then apply it to bite or sting.

- **Honey** is known for its healing abilities, so dab a little on the welt. The stickiness may even help stop you from scratching.

- **Vinegar** can be dabbed onto the welt or added to a bath. Pour 2 cups of vinegar into a tepid bath and relax in it for 20 minutes.

- **Basil** can be used in a poultice or as a tea wash. Crush the leaves with some water to make the poultice, which can be kept in place for 10 minutes before removing it. Alternatively, boil 2 cups of water and add 1/2 an ounce of dried basil. Allow the mixture to cool, and then use a clean washcloth to dab onto the affected areas.

- A **thyme** poultice with fresh leaves can be applied to the bite for 10 minutes.

- **Lemon balm** or even **echinacea** can also be used to make a poultice, as it can help reduce inflammation and prevent infection.

- Minced **garlic** in some petroleum jelly makes an excellent poultice. Leave the poultice in place for 10 minutes before washing it and placing a cool, moist cloth over the area to reduce itching. Repeat as needed. Don't add garlic directly to the bite, as it will burn.

- You can mix **peppermint, lavender**, or **tea tree essential oils** into a carrier oil that can be dabbed onto the bite, or a few drops can be added to your bath before you soak in it. It's also a great way to clear the sinuses. However, peppermint oil isn't suitable for young children.

- If you have some **chamomile** tea, add the bag to a cup of water and add it to the fridge to steep for 30 minutes. Remove the bag, squeeze the excess moisture out, and apply the bag to the bite for 10 minutes. Other herbal teas you can try include **peppermint** and **green** tea.

- **Witch hazel** extract can be dabbed onto each bite.

Generally, seeking medical assistance for a bug bite is rare. However, if you notice signs of infection you can't control, such as pus, fever, and red lines spreading beneath the skin (cellulitis), then it's best to see a doctor.

Minor Burns and Sunburn

There are three types of burns. First-degree burns, such as sunburn, usually result in red, swollen, hot, and painful skin. Second-degree burns are deeper burns that are red and splotchy, swollen, and sore, and blisters will likely develop. As long as the affected area is less than three inches, not in the face, and not in the joint of a limb, first and second-degree burns can be treated at home. However, if a young child or at-risk people are burned, it's best to take them to the hospital to ensure there aren't other potential injuries.

Third-degree burns are serious, and the depth of the burn can reach bone, also known as fourth-degree burns. With these burns, the skin is white or charred, and there is no pain due to the destruction of the nerves. Third and fourth-degree burns must be treated in the hospital to prevent infection.

Remedies

With first—and second-degree burns, the first course of action is to run cool water over the injury to stop the heat within the skin.

Keep the affected area under the water for 20 minutes or until the sting ends; it's vital to get the heat out before applying any remedy. To assist in treating the pain and inflammation, try some of the following remedies.

- **Aloe vera** gel is cooling, helps reduce scarring, and may assist in preventing blister development.

- **Manuka honey** may be expensive, all you need is a thin layer. It's known for its anti-inflammatory and antimicrobial properties.

- A **cold water compress** can be made by using a towel to soak up cold water and laying it on the affected area. *Don't rub the area!* This can cause the skin to separate. Use the compress for 5–15 minutes at a time, allowing the skin to dry between treatments.

- **Calendula** is a wonderful herb that can be used as a wash or a tincture to help with burns. A teaspoon of flowers steeped for 15 minutes in a cup of warm water creates a wash that can be used to make a compress once cool. Alternatively, use 1/2–1 teaspoon of calendula tincture in 1/4 cup water to make a compress.

- A **baking soda** bath is perfect for sunburn, while the poultice is perfect for a small burn area. Add a cup of baking soda to a tepid bath and relax in the water for 20 minutes. **Apple cider vinegar** can also be used in the same way to create a bath, or you can create compresses.

- The tannins from **black tea** are perfect for healing burned skin. Take 6 tea bags and steep them in 6 cups of boiling water for 10 minutes. Allow the tea to cool before making a compress with some material and then apply directly to the skin. Alternatively, a teabag of **chamomile** steeped in a cup of water will also make an effective compress.

- A spot of **milk** or **yogurt** in some water, applied with some cotton wool, is used by many to deal with sunburn.
- Grated **potato** is often used to help remove the heat from a burn and soothe the skin. Keep this poultice in place for 10 minutes.
- A compress with 3–4 tablespoons of **witch hazel** extract eases the inflammation of a burn. Recipe below.
- **Lavender**, either as an essential oil or as a dried herb, can be used to not only soothe the burn but also reduce stress and anxiety. Add 3–5 drops of essential oil to your bath, or up to 2 hands full of dried flowers in a mesh bag, before lounging in the bath water for 10–15 minutes.

Recipes

Witch hazel extract can be purchased or made. It's perfect to treat many skin ailments.

Witch Hazel Extract (Healey, n.d.)
Ingredients:

- 3 oz vodka
- 4 oz dried witch hazel bark
- 24 oz distilled water, extra set aside

Directions:

1. To a saucepan add 24 ounces distilled water with the witch hazel bark. Keep the temperature low and cover the saucepan. The mixture should be warm, but never simmer.

2. Allow the mixture to heat for an hour before straining.

3. Measure the volume of the witch hazel decoction and add that much water to it. If left with roughly 8 ounces of decoction, add 8 ounces of water and 3 ounces of vodka to make an 18% alcohol solution.

4. Pour into a clean container, seal it, label it, and store it in a cool, dry place until needed.

If the burn continues to be painful or becomes infected, it's best to see a doctor. While healing from sunburn, minimize your exposure to ensure you don't develop a worse burn or increase the risk of getting skin cancer.

Cuts and abrasions

Most cuts and abrasions can be dealt with at home as long as they're shallow. As long as you can stop the bleeding, remove any debris from the wound, and it's not too deep, you can treat these types of injuries. While it's unwise to add herbs to open wounds, once the injury has healed, there are many ways to speed up the recovery process.

Remedies

Even if you have had a deep cut that required stitching, the following remedies will assist in the healing process and reduce the chance of infection taking hold.

- **Aloe vera** has antimicrobial properties, so a thin layer of gel over an injury will fight possible infections. **Manuka honey** and **coconut oil** will give the same effect.

- There are several honey poultices you can try. The first is a poultice of **garlic and honey** or you can consider ground **cloves in honey**.

- A compress of **slippery elm bark** can be made by adding a teaspoon of powdered botanical to a cup of boiled water. Allow the liquid to cool before adding it to some cloth, and then apply it to the injury. You can also use **calendula** tea or the tincture diluted in water for the compress.

- **Turmeric** is well known for fighting pathogens and reducing inflammation. Add turmeric powder with just enough water to make a paste, and apply it to the injury with some gauze to keep it in place. Remove after a few hours and gently wash the area. Be warned, turmeric stains. The remedy can be reapplied after 4 hours.

- **Yarrow** has long been used to heal wounds in the field. The flowers and leaves can be mashed together to create a poultice. Leave the poultice in place for 30 minutes and wash the area well. Powdered, dried yarrow can also help stop bleeding.

- A fresh slice of **onion** helps fight potential bacterial infections in minor wounds.

- After enjoying a cup of **chamomile** tea to calm your nerves after an injury, apply the teabag to the injured area for 10 minutes to help reduce the pain. You can even add some dried **marigolds** to a tea bag and treat it the same, applying the cooled bag to the injury.

- Even essential oils have a place in helping wounds heal. **Lavender**, **tea tree**, or **peppermint** in coconut oil is a great way to introduce antibacterial and antimicrobial properties.

- When all else fails, a slice of fresh **cucumber**, will cool a minor wound and help reduce bleeding as cucumber has astringent (skin tightening) properties.

It's important to recognize when a wound is too much for you to handle at home. If you cannot get control over the bleeding, cannot remove debris from the wound, see fat or bone, or the injury is in the face or joint of a limb, it's best to have a doctor deal with it. Keep a close eye on possible spreading infection and deal with it with antibiotics if needed.

Poison Ivy and Rashes

Poison ivy, much like poison oak and poison sumac, contains a compound known as urushiol. When it comes into contact with the skin, it causes swelling, redness, itching, pain, hive-like bumps, and blisters. The plant oil is easily transferable, and it's possible to come into contact with urushiol through contaminated clothes or even your pet. The best way to treat this reaction is by avoiding it completely, but this isn't always possible.

Remedies

To prevent the reaction to poison ivy from getting worse, you need to get the urushiol off your skin. This can be done by running alcohol or washing the affected area with soap and water. While this will stop the reaction from getting worse, there may still be an initial reaction that can be treated with many different remedies. These remedies are also effective against rashes.

- **Baking soda** can be used as a paste for a small affected area, while a bath is best suited if a large area is affected. A cup is enough for a bath. Use 3 tablespoons of baking soda to a teaspoon of water for the paste.

- A poultice made from the stem and leaves of **jewelweed** can be applied to reduce the itchiness.

- To add a chilling effect and reduce itchiness, use the clear gel of **aloe vera**.

- Create a paste with a teaspoon of powdered **goldenseal** and some hot water, and apply it to the affected area with some cotton wool. Even drinking goldenseal tea will help the healing process from the inside out.

- A cup of **apple cider vinegar** and a 1/4 cup of cold water can be used to make a compress or a bath. However, some people may be too sensitive to having vinegar added to the poison ivy rash.

- One of the best soothing compresses that can be made for poison ivy rash is an **oatmeal** compress. Add a cup of oatmeal to a small bowl with enough water to cover the oatmeal. Allow it to steep for 10 minutes before straining the solids from the liquid. The oat "milk" can be applied to a cloth to make the compress, and the remaining oatmeal can be used as a poultice to reduce waste.

- Common fruits and vegetables can also remove the sting of poison ivy. **Cucumber**, **watermelon rinds**, and **banana peels** all assist in reducing the pain and itchiness. Perfect for that last use before being added to the compost.

- A cold water compress can be applied for 15–20 minutes several times throughout the day to help reduce the reaction.

- If you're close to the ocean, have a quick dip in the **salt water** to ease the symptoms of poison ivy. However, if you're nowhere close to an ocean, mix an ounce of salt in a quart of water and apply it to the affected area.

- **Tea tree** essential oil in your preferred carrier oil can be added to the rash to help lower the inflammation.

- Prevent the blisters and hives from weeping by adding some **witch hazel** extract. The astringent properties will help the skin to tighten and heal.

- **Oak bark** tea or bath will also be beneficial. To 4 cups of water, add 0.17 ounces of bark and bring to a boil. Strain the liquid and drink as needed. For the bath, add 0.7 ounces of the bark for 4 cups of water, strain, and then add the liquid to your bath. Alternatively, soak a cloth in the mixture and use it as a compress.

The only time a doctor will be needed for poison ivy is if a temperature of 100 °F or more develops, there's an allergic reaction, the face or eyes are affected, a large portion of the body is affected, or the bumps and blisters start to weep pus.

Bruises

Bruises, also known as contusions, occur when a bump or impact is hard enough to damage small blood vessels, causing blood to gather under the skin. The initial bruise is red, but in time, it will change to bluish-purple and, as it heals, to greenish-yellow. Bruises are unsightly for the most part, but unless you have an underlying issue or are on blood thinners, an injury resulting in a bruise isn't a major concern.

Remedies

No one likes to have a bruise visible all the time. Thankfully, many kinds of remedies can help the bruise heal faster.

- Creating a compress with cooled **lavender** or **chamomile** tea will help soothe the pain and can be reapplied every few hours. The 2botanicals are also known to help you relax.
- **Green and black tea** has a lot of tannins, which can help reduce bruising. Allow the tea bags to steep for a few minutes and add them to the bruise while still warm to let them do their magic.

- **Arnica** has been used for ages to deal with bruises. Either apply an arnica-infused oil to the affected area or create a dilution of the essential oil in your preferred carrier oil. *Don't* apply arnica to any broken skin.

- A cold **comfrey** compress can be made with a tablespoon of dried leaves to a quart of hot water. Allow the mixture to steep for 10–15 minutes before straining and allowing the mixture to cool in the fridge. Once adequately cooled, pour onto a cloth and apply to the affected area.

- **St. John's wort** can be used internally or externally. For tea, add 2 tablespoons of dried botanicals to a cup of hot water. Allow the mixture to steep for 20 minutes before drinking. Alternatively, dilute the essential oil with a carrier oil and apply it to the bruise.

- **Apple cider vinegar** can be used with the same volume of water to produce a compress that can be added to the bruise. Alternatively, soak a slice of onion in the vinegar for an hour before applying the slice to the bruise. For both methods, avoid adding to broken skin.

- Pineapple is high in **bromelain**, an enzyme that is anti-inflammatory, reduces pain and swelling, and also helps dissolve blood clots. Having more bromelain in your diet will help your body heal itself.

- **Heat and cold** treatments assist in many different ways but mostly help reduce inflammation, soothe pain, and get the blood flowing strongly again. For the **cold treatment**, take some ice (or a pack of frozen vegetables) and wrap it in cloth before applying it to the affected area for less than 10 minutes. Allow for a 20-minute break before repeating up to 3 times. For the heat **treatment**, you can use a hot water bottle on the bruise for 20 minutes before giving it a rest for an hour. An alternative to this is taking a hot bath.

- An **essential oil blend** of 5 drops of **calendula** oil, a drop of **cypress oil**, and 2 drops of **fennel oil** should be mixed well together with 4 teaspoons of your preferred carrier oil. Apply to the area as needed and rub gently.

- Another great essential oil is **rosemary**. Add 7 drops to the bath water and soak for at least 10 minutes. This can be combined with a heat treatment.

- **Aloe vera** can also assist in the healing process when rubbed into a bruised area.

While bruises aren't too much of a concern, under certain circumstances, they may be indicative of a deeper problem. If bruises appear for no reason, come and go in a short time, the pain and swelling are severe, the bruise covers a large area, affects the head, or prevents limbs from functioning, then it's time to discuss further steps with your doctor.

The point of first aid is to give the necessary care as quickly as possible. This not only prevents the injuries from getting worse but allows the healing process to start as soon as possible. While many other remedies can be used for a range of different first-aid-worthy ailments, take the time to discover which are more likely to happen to you and your family before learning obscure recipes that have ingredients that may be difficult to find.

If a specific ailment is more prevalent than others, this allows you the perfect opportunity to create remedies and store them away in your first aid kit. Remember that infused oils, salves, and dried tea blends can last a long time if properly stored. Take your time getting familiar with botanicals that aim to reduce pain (analgesic) and inflammation, fight infections (antimicrobial), and add some calm. Getting ill or injured is stressful, so don't neglect your emotions surrounding ailments. It doesn't help soothe the injury physically, but you're still stressed about it.

Now that you have a firm grasp on first aid remedies, it's time to look at remedies that can assist with cardiovascular health.

Chapter 7: Cardiovascular Remedies

The cardiovascular system—also known as the circulatory system—contains the heart, blood, and blood vessels. While a closed system, many outside influences can negatively affect it, leading to many different ailments that can become serious if ignored long enough. Stress, poor diet, and low activity are some of the main causes of illness that can affect the cardiovascular system.

High Blood Pressure

Normal blood pressure is 120/80 (systolic over diastolic), and anything higher than this is considered high blood pressure (hypertension) (*Best Home Remedies for Low Blood Pressure*, 2024). The higher the blood pressure, the higher the risk of damaging the organs (eyes, kidneys, and heart). There can also be an increased risk of memory loss, erectile dysfunction, strokes, and heart attacks.

Remedies

While high blood pressure can be dangerous if left unchecked, there are many remedies for dealing with it at home before a problem can occur.

- **Garlic** has a vasodilatory effect that lowers blood pressure and improves blood circulation. Crush a clove of garlic and soak it in 3.4 ounces of water for 6–8 hours. Drink on an empty stomach in the early morning.

- **Olive leaf** tea helps reduce blood pressure and has a calming effect. Add 2 tablespoons of ground, dried olive leaves, and steep in 2 cups of boiled water for 5–10 minutes. Strain and allow to cool before drinking. You can have up to 3–4 cups a day.

- **Blueberry juice** is high in antioxidants, which can help lower blood pressure when consumed daily. To a blender, add a cup of fresh blueberries, half a cup of water, and the juice of half a lemon. Blend until smooth and drink 1–2 times a day.

- **Hibiscus tea** contains anthocyanins that help decrease blood pressure. The darker the calyxes (lower part of the flower), the better. Add 0.035–0.07 ounces of hibiscus calyxes to a cup of boiled water. Steep for 5–10 minutes before straining. Drink 1–2 cups a day with at least eight hours between drinks. Don't have more than 0.2 ounces of dried flowers a day, as it may have toxic effects on some people. This tea can be a little sour, so don't be afraid to sweeten it with some honey.

- **Mangaba** tea is a vasodilator that helps lower blood pressure. Take 2 tablespoons of dried bark and add it to some freshly boiled water in a saucepan. Boil the mix for a few more minutes, remove from heat, and cover. Allow it to cool to room temperature before training and drink. Drink 2-3 cups daily.

- **Horsetail** is an invasive weed that can help lower blood pressure. Take 2–3 tablespoons of the dried leaves and add them to 2 cups of boiled water. Steep for 5-10 minutes before straining and drinking. Enjoy 2–3 times a day.

- **Valerian** tea creates a calming effect and helps reduce anxiety attacks that can drive blood pressure up. Add 1 teaspoon of dried valerian to a cup of boiled water and allow it to steep for 5-10 minutes. This herb may cause drowsiness, so drink a cup before bed. Can enjoy 2–3 cups a day.

- **Sweet basil** is not only tasty but also contains the antioxidant eugenol, which has many health benefits. You can either chew a few fresh leaves or create a tea by taking 3 tablespoons of dried basil along with 2 teaspoons of green tea and allowing them to steep in 2 cups of boiled water for 5–7 minutes. The tea can then be strained and sweetened.

- **Amla** or **Indian gooseberry** is best in the early morning as it can lower blood pressure by dilating blood vessels. Enjoy 1/2-1 teaspoon of alma powder in a cup of water. Alternatively, enjoy a cup of amla juice.

- **Cinnamon** can be enjoyed sprinkled over drinks or made into a paste with honey, which is a great way to sweeten drinks and reduce blood pressure. Mix 1/2 teaspoon powdered cinnamon with 1/2 teaspoon honey and add it to your preferred drink or 1/2 cup of warm water.

- **Ashwagandha** can assist in reducing blood pressure but should only be taken for a month and then not used for 3 months after. Add a teaspoon of dried root with a cup of water and allow the mixture to boil for 10 minutes before straining and drinking it.

- **Thyme** contains rosmarinic acid, which helps relax muscles and fight inflammation. Pick 8–10 springs and add them to a cup of boiled water. Allow the herb to seep for 10 minutes, and strain before drinking.

- Take a tablespoon of **celery seeds** and allow them to steep in boiled water for 10–15 minutes. After straining, enjoy hot or cold, with a slash of lemon or honey for flavor.

  Sesame and **flaxseeds** are also great for reducing blood pressure. Enjoy up to a tablespoon of sesame seeds or 4 tablespoons of flax seeds sprinkled over salads.

- **Ginger** is known to help with healthy circulation. Chop up a fresh root and take a tablespoon of the root to boil in a cup of water for 7–12 minutes before straining and enjoying hot. For more strength, add a stick of **cinnamon** to the boiling mixture.

- You can even enjoy a cup of **green tea**. A bag of green tea to a cup of boiled water is more than enough.

Some lifestyle changes that can assist with reducing blood pressure include quitting smoking and drinking excessively, getting more exercise and losing any extra pounds, managing stress, eating a whole food diet, reducing salt intake, and drinking water adequately for activity level.

If blood pressure reaches 180/120, it can be deadly, so ensure that you're communicating with your doctor if you're prone to high blood pressure or have a family history of high blood pressure.

Low Blood Pressure

When blood pressure reaches 90/60, it's considered low. Hypotension, or low blood pressure, is just as dangerous as having high blood pressure (*Best Home Remedies for Low Blood Pressure*, 2024). Those with this condition suffer from unexplained fainting (especially when standing up too quickly), dizziness, nausea, unexplained headaches, feeling weak, tired, sick, and confused.

Remedies

People rarely suffer from low blood pressure, but it isn't unheard of. Low blood pressure may be an indication of an underlying issue or can be caused by dehydration, medication, heart issues, and possible endocrine problems. While some of the remedies below are used to lower high blood pressure, they can also be used to help stabilize low blood pressure.

- **Tulsi (holy basil)** contains eugenol, the same as basil, but can assist with bringing blood pressure to normal levels. Consume 5–6 leaves on an empty stomach or make a tea. Take 1/2 a teaspoon of dried leaves, then add it to 1 1/2 cups water in a saucepan. Raise the temperature to medium, bring the mixture to a boil, and keep it there for 10–15 minutes. Strain and flavor with a teaspoon of lemon juice and honey.

- **Green tea** also helps to stabilize blood pressure.

- To create homemade **almond milk**, all you need to do is add 5–6 almonds to a glass of water and let them soak overnight. Remove the almonds and mash them into a paste before adding them to a cup of warm water or milk. Stir well before drinking. Enjoy the mixture daily.

- **Licorice** is a common remedy for low blood pressure. Licorice root contains glycyrrhizic acid, which affects fluid balance. Take an ounce of dried root and roughly chop it before adding it to a saucepan with 5 cups of boiled water. Continue to boil the water for another 10 minutes. Strain the mixture and enjoy with a dollop of honey.

A few lifestyle changes can help raise blood pressure. One is to consume smaller but more frequent meals or sprinkle a few raisins over your morning oatmeal. Raisins have high levels of potassium, which can help stabilize blood pressure.

Continual low blood pressure can lead to heart attacks, strokes, and kidney damage. However, low blood pressure can also be a sign of good health. If you are suffering from symptoms of low blood pressure and are not in good health, it's a good idea to discuss this with your doctor.

Cholesterol

There is a misconception that cholesterol is bad for the body. However, without cholesterol, the body wouldn't be able to make hormones, assist in making bile, or allow cells to perform their various functions. Cholesterol is made up of triglycerides, high-density lipoprotein (HDL, "good" cholesterol), and low-density lipoprotein (LDL, "bad" cholesterol) (*10 Home Remedies for High*

Cholesterol, n.d.). When eating a healthy diet, the body keeps the different cholesterol components in balance. However, due to genetics or poor diet, there can be an imbalance between HDL and LDL. When there are high levels of LDL, it can clog the arteries, resulting in strokes, heart attacks, and blood clots.

Remedies

Continuing to eat a diet high in fried foods and not enough omega-3 fatty acids can result in an imbalance in LDL. Thankfully, there are a few ways you can reduce your risks with some herbal remedies.

- Take 2 teaspoons of powdered **coriander seeds** (cilantro), then add it to a cup of boiled water and allow it to steep for a few minutes. After straining, you can drink it as is, add milk and honey, or add a teaspoon of seeds to a cup of boiling water, allowing it to steep for 2 minutes.
- **Amala** can be drunk daily, either as a glass of fruit juice or adding a teaspoon of the powder to a cup of boiled water.
- Improve your diet by adding 2 tablespoons of **flaxseed** sprinkled over oatmeal or salads.
- A tablespoon of **astragalus** root in 2 cups of water can be added to a saucepan before raising the temperature to bring the mixture to a simmer. You can drink this hot or cold after it has simmered for 10 minutes and been strained. Avoid this remedy if you're taking any immune suppressant or if taking lithium.

- Due to **garlic's** many benefits, it's often used as a cure-all. Eating 1–2 cloves a day, cooked or raw, is enough to gain all the benefits. However, if you get heartburn, consume less.

- **Green tea** is a great way to control cholesterol, but you should limit yourself to 6–8 cups daily.

- A teaspoon of **fenugreek seeds** can be soaked in a glass of water overnight and then transferred to a saucepan to boil until reduced by half. Strain the mixture and drink on an empty stomach. Alternatively, a tincture of **fenugreek leaves** can be made. Enjoy up to 3/4 teaspoon of the tincture 3 times a day with some water or under the tongue.

- **Yarrow** can also be used as a tea or tincture. Bring a cup of water with 1-2 teaspoons of dried leaves to boil. Boil for 10–15 minutes before straining and enjoying. Enjoy up to 3 cups a day. A tincture of yarrow can also be taken. Take 1/2–3/4 teaspoon daily.

- While mixing up a salad or when making a pasta salad, add up to 0.035 ounces of **tulsi**. Alternatively, eat it as-is.

- **Ginger** can also be eaten raw to help with cholesterol. You can enjoy up to 0.7 ounces of it a day.

- **Turmeric** can help reduce LDL. Mixing it with honey allows you to have a natural sweetener that can be added to any of your preferred drinks. Mix 1/3 cup of honey with 2 1/2 teaspoons of ground turmeric until well incorporated. Store the mixture in a cool area until ready to use it. Add a generous teaspoon mixture to your preferred drink with a pinch of black pepper to help absorption. Alternatively, add a teaspoon to a cup of boiled water with a dash of black pepper and lemon. A simple tea of 1/2 a teaspoon of ground powder can be added to a cup of warm water.

- To help reduce the risk of cardiovascular disease, add up to 0.35 ounces of powdered rosemary to food and drink daily.
- Another home remedy that people swear by is **apple cider vinegar**. This cure-all is also only a tablespoon required in a glass of warm water.

  However, not everyone enjoys the taste, so double the volume of water if the drink burns your throat.

The best way to deal with cholesterol is to give your body the nutrients and exercise it needs to create the environment required to bring balance to the body. A diet high in fiber, fruits, vegetables, and omega-3 fatty acids is ideal while improving activity, cutting back on drinking, and quitting smoking.

Before treating yourself with home remedies, be sure to determine your cholesterol level through a blood test.

Varicose Veins

Varicose veins, also known as spider veins, are swollen and unsightly veins that appear on the legs and feet. They may also be painful and itchy.

While these can develop due to age, they are also believed to be caused by pressure placed on the lower extremities or high blood pressure.

Remedies

While varicose veins are generally not a medical condition, there is a chance that complications can occur. These complications can cause blood clots and inflammation of the veins. With herbal remedies, the earlier you start treating, internally or externally, the better the chance of lowering the risk of complications.

- **Cayenne powder**, or any other chili powder, can help reduce varicose veins from the inside and outside. Cayenne pepper makes a wonderful addition to food, or you can enjoy up to a teaspoon of the powder in a cup of water up to 3 times a day. Alternatively, a salve can be made that can also help fight sinus pain, muscle aches, menstrual cramps, and arthritis. Recipe below.

- **Olive oil** is high in vitamin E, which makes it perfect for treating varicose veins. Gently rub the oil into the affected areas in small circular motions.

- You can even drink **apple cider vinegar** to promote healing. Depending on your taste, you can drink from 2 teaspoons up to 2 tablespoons in a glass of water twice a day. Alternatively, you can massage the vinegar undiluted into the varicose veins.

- **Grape seed extract** can be purchased over the counter but should be used as directed by a professional and never used when on blood thinners. Alternatively, try a **grapevine leaf** foot soak. Collect a cup of fresh leaves and boil them in 4 cups of water for 10–15 minutes before removing them from the heat and allowing them to cool until lukewarm. Pour the mixture, leaves and all, into a shallow basin while preparing another basin with cold water. Soak your feet in the grape leaf infusion for 5 minutes before placing your feet in the cold water for 10 seconds. Continue this cycle 3–4 times. Afterward, rub castor oil in a downward motion from the varicose veins to your feet, then lie down for a few minutes with your feet elevated.

- There are a range of essential oils that can also help. Add 3–5 drops of **lavender**, **sea pine**, **grapevine**, or **yarrow** to 3 tablespoons of your preferred carrier oil. The oil can be slightly warmed before massaging into the legs.

- If you don't mind the smell of **garlic**, it can also be used for a topical application. Slice 6 garlic cloves and place them in the juice of 3 oranges along with 2 tablespoons of olive oil. Give the mixture a shake after it steeps for 12 hours. Add a few drops to the inflamed veins and massage in small circles for 15 minutes. Cover the area with gauze, wrap it in place, and leave it overnight.

- Another over-the-counter supplement you can try is a **butcher's broom**. This supplement is also good for hemorrhoids.

- Add a few drops of **witch hazel extract** to a gauze and apply it to the area for 2–3 days for up to 2 months. Alternately, add 10–20 drops to a lukewarm bath and soak in it for 15 minutes. Also, use this treatment for up to 2 months.

- **Parsley,** with essential oils, **rose** and **marigold,** creates the perfect liquid extract to reduce varicose veins. Take a handful of fresh parsley and chop it finely before adding it to a saucepan with a cup of water. Boil the mix for 5 minutes. Steep the mixture until lukewarm before straining. Add a drop of each of the essential oils and place the mixture in the fridge until cool. Soak a cotton ball in the mixture and dab it on the affected area. Don't be afraid to consume parsley raw or add it to your juices or smoothies to have it work from the inside as well.

- **Marigolds** not only protect your garden but come with many other benefits, as long as you aren't allergic to them and you use edible varieties. **Calendula** is one of the edible species.

  Take up to a cup of fresh flowers, add it to 4 cups of water, and allow the mixture to boil for 5 minutes. Cool and strain the mixture, then soak it up with some gauze or cotton balls to add to the veins. Alternatively, sprinkle the flowers over your salads. They may be bitter, but that will also help with improving digestion.

- A poultice of fresh **ginger** can be applied to lower inflammation, or you can enjoy ginger tea.

- A 1/4 teaspoon dose of **pine bark** tincture, made with the bark and fresh sprigs of pine, will help you heal from the inside out.

Recipe

If you want a salve that can help with varicose veins, blocked sinuses, and muscle aches and pains, look no further than cayenne salve.

Cayenne Salve (de la Forêt, 2012)
Ingredients:

- 2 tbsp cayenne powder
- 1/4 c olive oil
- 1/2 oz beeswax

Directions:

1. Add the cayenne powder to the olive oil in a double boiler and warm it. It should just start to steam.
2. Remove the mixture from the heat and allow it to stand for 20 minutes.
3. Return the mixture to the heat and continue this cycle for at least an hour, though you can do more cycles.
4. Strain the oil through cheesecloth and return it to the cleaned double boiler.
5. Add the beeswax and heat over medium heat. Stir until the wax is melted and well incorporated.
6. Pour the salve into the waiting tins and allow to cool until solid.
7. Seal the tins, label them, and store them appropriately.

While herbal remedies can help, some lifestyle changes can complement them. Avoid wearing tight clothing and sitting cross-legged, get more exercise, raise your feet when you sit, and maintain a healthy weight.

Improving Heart Health

While the brain may be the most important organ, if it weren't for the heart, the brain wouldn't get the blood or nutrients it needs to function. A healthy heart allows you to live your life fully. A poor heart leaves you weak, short of breath, poor blood flow, and swollen lower limbs.

Remedies

High blood pressure and excess cholesterol are the biggest culprits of a weak heart. Many herbal remedies that can improve heart health are similar to those that combat high blood pressure and cholesterol.

- Consume at least 1 **garlic** clove a day. You can even sprinkle **cinnamon** over your usual drinks or breakfast cereals. **Cayenne** can also be added to your food, or you can add a 1/4 teaspoon of the powder to a cup of warm water.
- Alternatively, combine the anti-inflammatory properties of **cinnamon** with **turmeric**. In a saucepan, add 2 cups of milk, 1 tablespoon of honey, 1/4 teaspoon of ground cinnamon, and a teaspoon of ground turmeric. Simmer the mixture for 10 minutes and enjoy with a pinch of black pepper. This is known as golden milk.
- **Fennel** can be sprinkled over a salad to add a licorice twist or enjoyed as a tea. Take a teaspoon of fennel seeds and add

them to 2 cups of boiled water. Allow it to steep for a few minutes before straining and enjoying.

- Take 2 1/2 oz **dried hawthorn berries** and add them to 6 cups water in a saucepan. Bring the mixture to a boil before reducing to a simmer for 45 minutes. Remove from heat and strain. Hawthorn tea can be tart, so use some honey to combat this.

- If you're getting bored of dried **ginger**, mix it up by adding a few slices of fresh ginger to a cup of freshly boiled water. Allow it to steep for 5 minutes before fishing out the ginger and enjoying the tea. You can even add ginger slices to a freshly brewed cup of **green tea** to get additional benefits.

- **Coriander** leaves can be added to the diet if you like the taste, but it's not suited to everyone. Alternatively, take a cup of fresh leaves and chop them finely. Add the chopped leaves to a cup of boiled water and steep until the mixture is lukewarm. Strain and drink.

- **Olive leaf extract** can help lower blood pressure and is purchasable over the counter. A dose of 500–1,000 milligrams daily is generally safe.

- Teas don't need to be warm. Add 1/4 cup dried **hibiscus** to 4 cups cold water before stirring and refrigerating for at least 20 minutes, although overnight is better. Strain the mixture and serve with the preferred sweetener if it is too sour.

- **Ginseng tea** can be made with fresh or dried root. You will need 0.14–0.17 ounces of dried root (or 2–3 small roots, 1–2 medium roots, or 1 large root) per cup of hot water, which must be on the verge of boiling. Allow the mixture to steep for 5–10 minutes before straining and drinking. If using large roots, allow the steeping period to be longer.

Some of the best ways to keep your heart healthy are to improve your diet, get enough exercise, lower stress, go to yearly physicals with a medical professional, and listen to your heart.

Before taking an herbal remedy or supplement for your heart, it's important to discuss it with your doctor, as certain herbs—even those not taken for strengthening the heart—may trigger underlying cardiac conditions.

- **St. John's wort** interacts with many heart medications.
- **Hawthorn** may cause more problems than solve them, depending on the heart conditions.
- **Black cohosh** reacts to certain heart medications.
- High levels of **ginger** may be counterproductive and affect certain heart medications.
- **Ginko** is often used to boost energy, but it can affect warfarin and other medications with blood-thinning properties.
- **Saw palmetto** can thin the blood and reduce the effectiveness of clotting medication.
- **Evening primrose oil** can thin the blood and interact with certain heart medications.
- **Ginseng** interferes with anticoagulants and blood pressure.

- High levels of **garlic** can cause the blood to thin, but excessive amounts need to be eaten or too many supplements taken for this to occur.

When in doubt, always speak to your doctor to determine possible negative effects and interactions.

Many more cardiovascular herbal remedies can be used to strengthen your body, and it's your job to continue researching and finding them. In the next chapter, we'll look at different herbal remedies that can assist the brain.

Chapter 8: Neurological Remedies

Our brains are central to our identity and well-being, shaping who we are. However, they endure significant strain from our day-to-day activities, stressful jobs, and poor diets. This relentless pressure can cause exhaustion, anxiety, depression, insomnia, and migraines, among other issues.

Headaches and Migraines

Headaches and migraines can make life difficult. While some can start small and irritating, others can be debilitating, leading some people to have to hide in a dark and quiet room to prevent excess pain.

Remedies

While some headaches and migraines can be triggered by hormonal changes, blocked sinuses, diet, and even dehydration, the quicker they are dealt with, the better. Many remedies can be used to treat a headache or migraine, some of which can be carried on your person.

- In the previous chapter, it was noted that **cayenne** can help with pain. Applying the cayenne salve to your temples will help relieve a headache. Alternatively, add 1/4 teaspoon powder to warm water and use a cotton bud to apply the mixture to your nostrils, where you can breathe in the smell.

- A teaspoon of dried **butterbur root** can be turned into an infusion or tea to soothe an aching head. For the infusion, add the root to a cup of water and allow it to steep for 10–12 hours before straining and drinking. To make the tea, add the root to a cup of water. Once it is boiling, lower the temperature and simmer for 3-5 minutes. Afterward, strain the liquid and enjoy.

- Contrary to its name, **feverfew** doesn't fight fevers well but is a better headache reliever. Use a teaspoon dried or 3 teaspoons fresh in a cup of boiled water. Steep the mixture in a covered cup for 5-15 minutes. Strain and enjoy 1–3 cups a day. Alternatively, you can eat a few leaves, but they are very bitter.

- **Peppermint** can be used as a tea or an essential oil. The essential oil can be smelled or added to a carrier oil and applied to the temples. For tea, use 1/2 a cup of dried leaves to 3–4 cups of water that's just reached boiling temperature. Allow the leaves to steep in the hot water for 5 minutes. Strain the mixture and enjoy the tea, breathing deeply to inhale the essential oils. Peppermint-infused oil can also be used to make salves.

- **Lemon balm**, related to peppermint, can also assist in breaking headaches. Create a tincture using 3 parts dried lemon balm with 2 dried parts feverfew, topping up with 100 proof alcohol of choice. Steep for 2–6 weeks in a warm and sunny location, shaking the container daily. After straining, use 1/4–1/2 teaspoon once the symptoms start, and continue to take another dose every 30–60 minutes until the pain stops.

- Another blend to consider is made with 1 part feverfew, 1 part **chamomile**, , 2 parts **skullcap**, and 2 parts lemon balm. All the herbs should be fresh to make this tea. Weigh the herbs, add the same weight of boiled water, and allow the mixture to steep for 30–60 minutes. Drink 1/4 cup upon the start of the headache, and continue to drink this dose every 30 minutes until the headache disappears.

- **Willow bark** is why we have aspirin, which is still an effective pain medication. Put 2 teaspoons of the dried bark into a cold cup of water. Bring the water to a boil and let it boil for 10 minutes. Remove from heat and steep for 30 minutes. This mixture is bitter and astringent, so add 1/2 a teaspoon of honey per cup. Avoid this remedy if you are on blood thinners or if you have gastrointestinal issues.

- **Valerian** can be used as a tincture or tea. Don't exceed 1–1 1/2 teaspoons of the tincture a day. For the tea, add a teaspoon of the dried root to a cup of boiled water, then allow it to steep for 5–10 minutes before straining and drinking.

- **Ginger** can be added to food, or add a teaspoon of ground ginger to a cup of boiled water. Allow it to steep for a few minutes before straining and drinking.

- Add a tablespoon of **coriander seed** to 2 cups water and bring to a boil for 2 minutes. Remove from the heat and allow it to steep for 10 minutes. Strain and sip the drink throughout the day. Coriander or cilantro should be avoided if you are allergic to anise, fennel, caraway, or dill.

- **Lavender** has long been used to treat headaches. Once in a carrier oil, it can be dabbed on the temples, or the essential oil can be inhaled. **Rosemary** essential oil can be applied the same way.

- **Linden** not only helps with clearing a headache but also lowers blood pressure and anxiety, promoting sleep. Use a tablespoon of dried blossoms or 2 tablespoons of fresh blossoms in a cup of boiling water. Allow the mixture to steep for 15 minutes or more if you'd like it to be stronger. Strain and then enjoy with some lemon or honey.

- A poultice of **horseradish** applied to the forehead is said to break headaches. Alternatively, create a poultice of **mullein** leaves.

- **Honeysuckle** is a light tea best made with fresh, slightly bruised flowers. Use 1 part flowers to 2 parts cold water, then allow the mixture to steep in the fridge for 6–8 hours. Enjoy once strained.

- A 1/4 teaspoon **yarrow** tincture will help with the pain.

- **Teaberry**, also known as **wintergreen**, tincture is perfect for adults but is best avoided for children. Take a cup of fresh leaves to a cup of quality vodka. Ensure the leaves are under the alcohol level before storing the container for up to 6 weeks in the dark. Strain and take up to a teaspoon when the headache starts.

- **Chamomile** grows easily in the garden, and all you need is 3–4 tablespoons of fresh flowers to a cup of boiling water. Steep for only 5 minutes, or the mixture will be too bitter.

- **Turmeric** helps combat inflammation, so try the golden milk recipe in Chapter 7.

- **Boswellia**, also known as **frankincense**, is perfect for cluster headaches. Use 0.035–0.25 ounces of resin in 2 cups of hot water (140–176 °F) and stir until dissolved. The resin can also be chewed.
- **Passionflower** eases tension, promotes calmness, and is safe for children. Add 1–2 teaspoons of dried passionflower in a cup of boiled water and cover. Allow it to steep for 20–30 minutes. Drink 1/2 a cup up to 4 times a day.

Recipes

Headache Blend Balm (Joybilee Farm, n.d.)
Ingredients:

- 2 ½ tbsp beeswax
- 5 drops lavender essential oil
- 20 drops eucalyptus essential oil
- 1 tsp dried lavender blossoms, or 1 tbsp fresh
- 2 tbsp shea butter
- 15 drops rosemary essential oil
- 50 drops peppermint essential oil
- 1 tsp dried peppermint leaves or 1 tbsp fresh
- 4 tbsp olive oil
- 1 tsp dried lemon balm leaves or 1 tbsp fresh

- 15 drops cajuput (cajeput) essential oil

Directions:

1. If using fresh herbs, allow them to wilt for 12 hours before use.
2. Add the olive oil to a double boiler and simmer gently for an hour to create an infused oil with the herbs.
3. Remove from the heat and allow to cool until it can be handled safely.
4. Strain the oil through a fine mesh or cheesecloth, squeezing all excess oil from the mixture.
5. Clean the double boiler and return the infused oil before adding the shea butter and beeswax. Continue to heat until the wax and butter melts.
6. Stir the mixture with a wooden skewer until everything is well incorporated.
7. Remove the mixture from the heat and let it cool for a few minutes before adding the essential oils. Keep stirring to distribute the oils throughout the mixture.
8. Pour the completed mixture into the prepared tins and cool until solid.
9. Add the lids, seal the tins, label them, and store them in a cool, dry area.
10. Apply to temples.

Some alternative therapies for headaches and migraines include acupressure, acupuncture, yoga, massage, getting quality sleep, and increasing magnesium intake.

If headaches and migraines are affecting your ability to work or live normally, it's time to discuss other treatments with your doctor.

Fighting Insomnia

Sleep is vital for the body; it's the time when healing and restoration occur. It's also the only time the brain can truly rest. If you don't get enough sleep, it can have a cascading effect on your body. Poor-quality sleep, especially for an extended period, increases the risk of many diseases and can also lead to stress, anxiety, and depression.

Remedies

It's recommended that people should get 7–9 hours of sleep a night. However, many people struggle to sleep for a variety of reasons, some of which can be addressed by taking certain herbal remedies. Ideally, these remedies should be taken 30–60 minutes before settling into bed. Try some of the following to get you back into the correct sleeping pattern.

- Try **valerian root** and **passionflower** tea. Alternatively, try the **ashwagandha** tea from Chapter 7 or the moon milk recipe below.

- **Lemon balm** tea can be made by adding a teaspoon of dried leaves (or 5–6 fresh leaves) to a cup of boiled water, allowing it to steep for 5–10 minutes.

- A teaspoon of dried **hops** in a cup of hot water, steeped for 7 minutes. Don't use if suffering from any hormone-related conditions.

- **Black cohosh** works particularly well for menopausal women suffering from insomnia. If taking a tincture, the dose is 1/2–3/4 teaspoons daily. To make a tea add 0.7 ounces to 34 ounces of water, and bring to a boil. Lower to a simmer for 20–30 minutes, or until the mixture is reduced by a third. Drink a cup 3 times a day. The mixture will last 48 hours in the fridge.

- A warm **hibiscus** tea will help you relax before bed. Take 1/3 cup of dried flowers and add them to 2 cups of boiled water. Steep for at most 5 minutes before enjoying with some honey or lemon.

- While **elderberry** is more commonly used to treat colds, it can also assist in sleep. Take a tablespoon of dried berries and add them to 2 cups water. Bring the mixture to a boil, then simmer for 15–20 minutes. You can also add a stick of **cinnamon** or 1/4 teaspoon of the ground spice.

- For sleep, a weaker **chamomile** tea is needed, compared to one that treats a headache. Take a teaspoon of dried chamomile and steep it for 5 minutes in a cup of boiled water.

- Essential oils such as **lavender** and **peppermint** beckon sleep. Peppermint tea will also help to calm the nerves before sleep. Take a teaspoon of dried leaves and steep in 6 ounces of hot water for 6 minutes. Be sure to breathe in the fumes as you enjoy your drink.

- A cup of **holy basil** made with a teaspoon of dried herb in a cup of hot water, steeped for a few minutes with beckon sleep. This herb can also be combined with chamomile.

- **St. John's wort** essential oil can be applied to temples before sleep, or tea can be made. Add a teaspoon of the dried herb to a cup of boiled water and allow it to steep for 15–30 minutes covered. Enjoy 2–3 cups for up to 6 weeks.

- **Skullcap** can be used either as a tincture or tea. The tincture dose is roughly 30 drops 3–4 times a day at mealtimes and an hour before bed. Alternatively, make tea using a tablespoon of dried skullcap to 2 cups of boiled water. Steep for 10 minutes and sweeten as needed.

- Gather a 1/4 cup of dried **magnolia** bark and allow it to soak in 8 cups of cold water for 30 minutes. Then bring the mixture to a boil and lower to a simmer for 30–120 minutes, enough to reduce the liquid to 2 cups. This is a bitter and astringent drink, so sweeten it if needed.

- Add 1 tsp dried **kava kava** to 1 cup of water and blend until well incorporated. The drink may numb your mouth, so don't be alarmed.

- Take 1–2 teaspoons of dried **California poppy** (leaves and flowers) and add to a cup of boiled water. Allow it to steep for 10 minutes. Alternatively, you can add 1/2 a teaspoon of California poppy tincture to water or tea.

- A cup of **tart cherry** juice.

- A tincture or tea made with **vervain**, also known as **verbena**. The tincture dose is 1–2 teaspoons. For the tea, add 1–2 teaspoons of dried herb and allow it to steep in a pint of boiled water for 10–15 minutes. Enjoy up to 3 cups a day.

Recipes

Try some of the following recipes to send you off to la-la land.

Moon Milk (La Forge, 2019)
Ingredients

- 1/4 tsp ground ginger
- 1 tsp sweetener of choice (honey or maple syrup)
- 1 c milk or milk alternative of choice
- 1/2 tsp ground ashwagandha powder
- 1/2 tsp ground cinnamon
- 1 tsp coconut oil
- a pinch of ground nutmeg

Directions:

1. Pour the milk into a saucepan and bring it to a low simmer.
2. Add the ground herbs and whisk until well incorporated.
3. Continue to gently simmer for another 5 minutes.

4. Remove from the heat and pour the moon milk into a waiting cup before stirring in the coconut oil and preferred sweetener.

Sleepy Time Tincture (Wells, 2021)
Ingredients:

- 2 c 80-proof or stronger vodka
- 1 tbsp dried hops flowers
- 2 tbsp dried yarrow flowers
- 2 tbsp dried chamomile flowers
- 1 tbsp dried stevia leaf
- 1 tbsp dried peppermint leaf
- 2 tbsp dried catnip
- 2 tbsp dried oat straw

Directions:

- Add all the herbs to a clean container and pour the alcohol over the top, leaving 1–2 inches of headspace.
- Seal the container and leave it in a cool, dark place for 2–8 weeks (depending on the strength you want), shaking daily.
- Strain the mixture through some cheesecloth and store the tincture in a dark tincture bottle.
- Label the bottle appropriately and keep it in a cool, dark place.

- For adults, take 2–3 droppers full, while children can have up to 1 dropper full per day.

Sleepy Time Tea (Penrod, n.d.)
Ingredients:

- 8 fresh rose petals
- 2 tbsp fresh chamomile buds or 2 tsp dried
- 1 tbsp fresh peppermint
- 1 tbsp fresh lavender buds or 1 tsp dried
- 1 tbsp lemon balm
- 2–3 c boiled water.

Directions:

1. Add the boiled water to a bowl or French press with all the herbs.
2. Allow the mixture to steep for 12 minutes, then press the French press's plunger down or strain the liquid using cheesecloth.
3. The recipe makes 2 cups. Enjoy a cup before bed and store the other in the fridge until the next day.

Combining these remedies with good sleep hygiene is the best cure for overcoming insomnia, but you can make other lifestyle changes. Try getting more exercise during the day and not consuming large meals too close to going to sleep. Alternatively, try meditation or adding melatonin supplements. If none of the lifestyle changes or supplements help, and insomnia starts to affect your daily life, it's time to see a doctor.

Relieving Anxiety and Stress

Everyone experiences anxiety or stress at some point in their lives. Some manage it better than others. If anxiety isn't dealt with early enough, it can develop into stress. With long periods of anxiety and stress, the body feels like it's constantly in fight or flight mode, increasing blood pressure and heart rate and causing damage to organs over time. In time, it'll affect your will to want to do anything.

Remedies

While anxiety and stress are normal, constantly remaining in these states is not healthy. You can try many lifestyle changes, techniques, and herbal remedies to alleviate the problems you may be experiencing. Try some of the following.

- An **ashwagandha** tincture will help lower cortisol, the stress hormone. Take up to 90 drops twice daily. Another tincture you can try is hemp-derived **cannabidiol** (CBD). This type of CBD contains less than 0.3 % tetrahydrocannabinol (THC) and can be found in gummy sweets and tinctures at many pharmacies. A standard tincture dose is about 30 drops.

- Some teas that can assist include **valerian**, **chamomile**, **passionflower**, **lemon balm**, and **kava kava**. All recipes can be found in earlier sections of this chapter.

- Aromatherapy has been used for ages to help alleviate the symptoms of stress and anxiety. Some of the best essential oils to soothe anxiety include **lavender**, **ylang-ylang**, and **clary sage**. You can also use **bergamot** and **grapefruit**. However, these essential oils are photosensitive and can cause a burn when exposed to the sun. Apply the essential oils in their carrier oil to the inside of the wrist or the neck. Alternatively, smell the essential oils directly from their bottles.

Some lifestyle changes and techniques that may assist in fighting anxiety include exercise, reducing smoking and drinking, meditation, and adding a weighted blanket to your bed to help improve sleep.

If your anxiety is chronic (more than six months) and you are suffering from symptoms such as digestive issues, chronic fatigue, increased heart rate, and difficulty sleeping, it may be time to consider speaking to a doctor. This is especially true if you suddenly find yourself pulling back from friends and family, no longer enjoying your hobbies, or are considering self-harm.

Mood Shifts

No one reason causes depression. For some people, it could be due to unbalanced hormones; for others, it's trauma (fresh or old), chronic illness, and many other reasons. Depression causes a lower quality of life where people feel trapped with no way out. Those suffering from chronic conditions may find their symptoms are worse during this time. Sadly, if depression is treated, there is an increased risk of self-harm or even suicidal thoughts.

Remedies

There are different levels of depression, some of which can be dealt with through lifestyle changes, therapy, and even herbal remedies. Mild to moderate depressive symptoms can be treated with herbal remedies, but in the case of severe depression, it's best to have trained professionals work with you to improve your life.

- **St. John's wort** can be used as a tea or a tincture to treat mild depression. A professional best determines the dose used, as this herb can interact with antidepressant medication, worsening depression.

- **Ginseng** (*Panax* genus specifically) can help with stress-related depression. Boil a cup of water and allow it to cool for 2–3 minutes before adding a tablespoon of powdered root. Allow the mixture to steep for 5 minutes before drinking.

- Boost your moods with teas that include **chamomile**, **ashwagandha**, **valerian root**, and **kava kava**. **Maca root** powder can be added to any of these teas to bolster their effects. Add 2–3 teaspoons of the powder to a warm cup of water or tea and stir until it's dissolved. Straining is necessary.

- Aromatherapy using oils such as **lavender**, **thyme**, **rosemary**, **valerian**, **jasmine**, **chamomile**, **bergamot**, **holy basil**, **sweet basil**, **rose**, **lemon balm**, and **geranium** helps boost mood.

- **Ginkgo** or **ginkgo biloba** can be purchased as supplements over the counter, or you can make a tea. Take an ounce of dried leaves and steep for 10 minutes in 2cups of boiled water.

- ***Rhodiola rosea*** **(golden root)** is a wonderful herb that helps against stress. Place a tablespoon of dried root into a cup of boiled water and let it steep for 12-15 minutes. You can have 1–2 cups per day.

- Generally, when using **thyme**, you don't need much more than what you would normally put in food. The herb contains natural lithium, which helps alleviate depression. A tea can be made with several sprigs added to a cup of boiled water. Allow the herbs to steep for 5–8 minutes before drinking.

Due to the different ways that depression can be caused, there are many alternatives to treating it. An improved diet with more fruits, vegetables, fish, nuts, seeds, and foods high in magnesium, such as avocado, will help. Getting exercise for at least 15 minutes up to 3 times a week will also be beneficial.

Self-care, meditation, yoga, and acupuncture can also assist. It's also important to reduce depressants from your life, such as alcohol and drugs; even cutting coffee out will help. Even light therapy has been beneficial to those who suffer from seasonal affective disorders (S.A.D.), especially during winter.

As with anxiety, if you start feeling that you no longer enjoy life, friends, family, and hobbies, it may be in your best interest to talk to your doctor about therapies and other medications that will improve your outlook.

Depression can be a dark hole, and there is no reason for you to suffer it without help. Even speaking to someone can brighten your day a little.

Mental-Emotional Well-Being

Perhaps you're not fully in the grips of anxiety, stress, or depression, but you want to prevent these conditions from affecting you by strengthening yourself against their development. It's vital to have good mental-emotional well-being, as this forms part of your whole being and is sadly ignored in favor of just treating the body.

Remedies

The following remedies are perfect for guarding against exam stress, mentally preparing for interviews, and even protecting against stressors such as illness or worse.

- Some teas you can try, recipes found within this and previous chapters, include **St. John's wort**, a**shwagandha**, **lemon balm**, **passionflower**, **chamomile**, **kava kava**, **linden**, **ginseng**, or **tulsi**.

- **Motherwort** assists in lowering anxiety, and depressive symptoms while improving sleep, concentration, and memory. Take a cup of dried leaves and flowers (or 3 cups fresh) and a quart of boiled water. Add the herb to and cover, allowing the mixture to steep for 15–30 minutes. Enjoy a cup 3 times a day. Alternatively, 1/2–1 teaspoon tincture 3 times a day.

- **Albizia**, a type of mimosa tree, helps alleviate insomnia, depression, and anxiety and is often used in traditional Chinese medicine. The dosage should be determined by a professional, as health, age, and other conditions can play a role in how this herbal remedy may affect you.

- Some essential oils that can improve mental-emotional well-being include **peony**, **rose**, **rosemary**, and **tulsi**. The best rose species to use are *Rosa damascena* and *R. contifolia*.

- Herbal additions to food that can assist include **rosemary**, **saffron**, and **tulsi**. Consuming more **oats** in your diet, along with herbal remedies, will also help lower anxiety and mild depression.

Whether fighting anxiety or depression, it's important to realize that herbal remedies aren't miracle cures. It's important to get to the root cause of the problem, whether spiritual, mental, emotional, or physical. Herbal remedies only help to strengthen the body to give it a fighting chance.

Reviewing your life and making some changes for the better is a good idea. Find or return to a loved hobby, connect with friends and loved ones, practice relaxation techniques, reconnect with nature, get some fresh air, improve sleep hygiene, and monitor how you feel on good versus bad days. There is no need for large, immediate changes. Daily small changes are good enough to build up resistance to stressors. Don't forget to do some self-care and know when to step back from a stressful situation, especially if you can't control what may happen.

Now that you have managed to fortify your mind, it's time to fortify your gut in the following chapter.

Chapter 9: Gastrointestinal Remedies

The gastrointestinal tract starts at the mouth and ends at the anus, making it the longest organ system in the body. Every part plays a role in physically and chemically breaking down food, absorbing what is needed, and excreting what isn't.

When working well, you are hardly aware of the organs that work to digest your food. However, when something goes wrong, you quickly become painfully aware of these organs and suffer from problems such as bloat, diarrhea, constipation, nausea, vomiting, and more—not to mention that poor digestion puts you at risk of nutrient deficiency.

Bloating and Constipation

Bloating is when excess gas builds up in the digestive tract. This can be caused by the types of food and drinks consumed, eating too fast, overeating, swallowing air, or constipation.

Constipation is an infrequency of bowel movements, usually three times or less a week. There are various reasons this can occur, including a poor diet, dehydration, stress, not getting enough fiber, or not listening to the body's natural cues to have a bowel movement.

In some cases, chronic diseases (such as irritable bowel syndrome, IBS), certain medications, and low activity can also have an impact on bowel movements.

Remedies

As constipation is one of the reasons bloating can occur, many home remedies seek to deal with bloating in conjunction with constipation, helping to alleviate symptoms from both discomforts.

- Many teas from the previous chapters not only help calm nerves but also the digestive tract. Try teas such as **ginger**, **lemon balm**, **fennel**, **chamomile**, **turmeric** (or golden milk), **elderberry**, and **black tea** to reduce constipation and ease the symptoms of bloating. **Peppermint** essential oil in a carrier oil can also be rubbed on the abdomen.
    - Chamomile tea is particularly good against bloating caused by *Helicobacter pylori,* a bacteria that can cause ulcers.
- **Peppermint** tea can be combined with **wormwood** tea, as it's bitter and astringent. Take 1/2–1 teaspoon of dried wormwood and steep it in a cup of boiled water for 5–15 minutes. The longer you steep, the more bitter it'll be. Avoid adding sweeteners, as bitter drinks are often associated with aiding digestion.
- The bitter-sweet tea of **gentian root** is ideal for relieving bloat but shouldn't be used if you have an ulcer. Steep 1–2 teaspoons of dried root in a cup of boiled water for 3–10 minutes.
- **Angelica root** is another bitter tea that can be combined with lemon balm to improve its taste. In a saucepan containing 2 cups of freshly boiled water, add a teaspoon of dried root, reduce the heat, and simmer for 15-20 minutes.

Remove from the heat and let sit for 5 minutes. Avoid this remedy if you are on blood thinners.

- Chewing on one **betel** leaf after a meal will help reduce constipation and bloating.

- **Ajwain** seeds can also be chewed after a meal, or a teaspoon can be added to a cup of hot water and steeped for 5 minutes before drinking.

- As long as you don't have stomach ulcers or gastritis, **cardamom** tea can be enjoyed before a meal. Add a teaspoon of seeds to a cup of freshly boiled water, allowing it to steep for at least 10 minutes.

- A teaspoon of **star anise** seeds (approximately 2 pods) in a cup of boiled water should be allowed to steep for 5–10 minutes before drinking. Enjoy 2–3 cups daily as long as you're over 12 years old.

- **Cumin** is a fragrant spice. If you want it to work for constipation, take a teaspoon of the seeds and roast them over heat until their scent is noticeable. Add the seeds to a cup of water and boil for 1–2 minutes. This must be drunk warm.

- **Buckthorn** has a laxative effect but shouldn't be used as a long-term remedy, as it can lead to mild to acute liver failure. Add 0.07 ounces of finely chopped dried buckthorn to 2/3 cup of boiled water and allow it to steep for 5–10 minutes.

- **Slippery elm** is a particularly good herbal remedy for constipation caused by IBS. Add 1–3 teaspoons of powdered slippery elm to a cup of water and drink up to 3 times daily.

- **Aloe vera juice** is lauded as a great remedy for constipation. However, not everyone can stomach the bitterness, so be wary. Enjoy up to a cup after each meal.

Recipe

While aloe vera juice can be purchased, it can contain additives you'd rather not consume. Here is an easy-to-follow recipe to make it at home.

Aloe Vera Juice (Delio, 2021)
Ingredients:

- 1/2 large aloe vera leaf
- 1 qt water
- 2 tbsp honey or agave (optional)
- juice of 2 limes (optional)

Directions:

1. Remove the outer green of the leaf, retaining the clear gel.
2. If you notice yellow liquid on the clear gel, wash it under cool water.
3. Chop the gel roughly and add it to the blender with the remaining ingredients.
4. Process to the consistency of choice.
5. Do a taste test, and add more lime or sweetener as needed.

6. The juice will last in the fridge for up to a week.

Alongside the herbal remedies, there are some lifestyle changes you can benefit from. Improve your diet by including more fiber (such as psyllium husk, prunes, and rhubarb), reduce dairy intake if you are intolerant or sensitive, add more pre- and probiotics, and enjoy some coffee to get the intestines working harder. Don't forget to hydrate and include some light activity.

Seek medical treatment if constipation lasts longer than three weeks, there is blood in the stool, or you have severe abdominal pain.

Diarrhea

Diarrhea is loose, watery bowels that occur three times or more in a day. This ailment can be caused by diseases, bacteria, parasites, poor quality or contaminated food, or consuming food that you're sensitive to. Normally, symptoms are acute, lasting no more than 2days. This leads to dehydration, which needs to be addressed quickly. When diarrhea is chronic, lasting up to four weeks or more, it's likely due to a chronic disease such as IBS.

Remedies

- Tea is a great way to hydrate yourself and replace any lost salts. Try herbal teas such as **ginger**, **chamomile**, **peppermint**, and **slippery elm**.

- If you don't mind bitters, a type of tincture usually made with bitter ingredients, try some artichoke leaf bitters. Recipe below.
- Due to the tannins found in berry leaves, the leaves of **blackberries**, **blueberries**, and **raspberries** are often used to reduce the severity of diarrhea. Try 7–10 fresh raspberry leaves (or a teaspoon of dried leaves to 2–3 dried raspberries) in a cup of boiled water. Allow the mixture to steep for 5 minutes.
- If you live in tropical regions, you may have lemongrass growing in your garden. Roughly chop enough leaves to fill 2 cups and add to a saucepan with 4 cups of freshly boiled water. Allow the mixture to boil for a further 5 minutes, then bring the temperature down to simmer for another 5 minutes.

Recipe

Bitters are known to help with gastrointestinal issues, so give this artichoke bitters a chance to change your life.

Artichoke Bitters (Alieta, 2017)
Ingredients:

- 12 oz organic vodka (80 proof)
- 1 tbsp dried artichoke leaf
- 1 tbsp dried cardamom pods

- 1 tbsp dried orange peel

Directions:

1. Add all the ingredients to a container large enough to hold 12 ounces of vodka and maintain a 1–2 inches headspace.
2. Store in a cool, dry area for up to 2 weeks, shaking daily. For a weaker bitter, allow the mixture to steep for 3 days.
3. Strain and transfer the liquid into half-ounce amber containers with a dropper.
4. Add 1–2 droppers worth of bitters in a cup of tea or soda water to make it more palatable.

When suffering from diarrhea, it's important to stay hydrated and eat light meals containing bland foods. The BRAT diet (banana, rice, apple sauce, and toast), along with clear soups and broth, saltine crackers, and plain potatoes, should be consumed for the next 24–48 hours.

Afterward, return to your regular diet, reducing your intake of fatty foods and taking in more pre and probiotics.

Diarrhea is serious, and if it lasts longer than 48 hours (24 hours for a child), it's best to approach a doctor for assistance. This is also true if a fever over 102 °F accompanies diarrhea, the stool is bloody or has a tar consistency, pus is present in the stool, or there is severe dehydration.

Diarrhea is more than the loss of water; it's also the loss of vital electrolytes (mineral salts). These need to be replaced, so add electrolyte replacers during your recovery.

Stomachache

When suffering from digestive issues (such as constipation, bloat, indigestion, and diarrhea), you may deal with a stomachache. This pain can also be triggered by certain antibiotics (which is why some state that they should be taken after a meal) and acid reflux.

Remedies

In most cases, stomachaches can be dealt with in the comfort of your own home with the following remedies.

- Drink teas containing **ginger**, **peppermint**, **sweet basil,** or **chamomile**. You can also try drinking **ginger ale** or **aloe vera juice** or eating **peppermint candies**. You could also consider eating **figs** to ease a stomach ache. However, avoid this if you have diarrhea.
- A tablespoon of **apple cider vinegar** combined with a teaspoon of honey in a cup of warm water can soothe a stomachache.
- Mix a 1/4 teaspoon of **baking soda** in 4 ounces of warm water.
- There are a range of bitters that can assist in easing stomach aches. Try 1–2 droppers of **peppermint**, **fennel**, **ginger**, or **cinnamon** bitters.
- **Licorice** tea can also be drunk as long as you don't have

- high blood pressure. For a stomachache, take 1–2 teaspoons of powdered root and add it to a cup of boiled water, allowing it to steep for 5 minutes.

If suffering from a stomachache, it's a good idea to use the BRAT diet and avoid eating fatty or spicy foods.

Issues with the digestive tract aren't the only cause of stomachaches. Ovarian cysts, kidney stones, appendicitis, and more can also cause abdominal pain. It's important to know your body to determine if you're suffering from a digestive issue or something more serious. If the pain lasts longer than a week, becomes severe, or prevents you from functioning, it's time to speak to your doctor.

Other symptoms to be on the lookout for include vomiting blood or what appears to be coffee grounds, severe constipation, chest pain, difficulty breathing, jaundice, or tar-like or bloody stool.

Indigestion and Acid Reflux

Indigestion and acid reflux go hand-in-hand but aren't the same thing. Indigestion tends to affect the stomach, while acid reflux is when stomach acid travels up the esophagus. These ailments can lead to many problems, including gastritis, excess burping or flatulence, bloating, ulcers, and a burning feeling behind the breastbone or upper stomach.

Remedies

Diet generally causes indigestion and acid reflux, but there is no reason to suffer from them. If you know a particular food triggers them, cut that food from your life. If you don't know what is causing them, here are a few remedies to help soothe the burn.

- Many teas that help soothe other digestive issues can be used to treat indigestion and acid reflux. Try **peppermint**, **chamomile**, **ginger**, **fennel seed**, **licorice root**, **turmeric** (or golden milk), **lemon balm**, and **cinnamon tea**.
    - For indigestion, take 1/2 teaspoon of crushed **fennel seeds** and add them to a cup of boiled water, allowing them to steep for 10 minutes before drinking. Alternatively, eat a teaspoon of the seeds.
    - Be wary of taking peppermint oil or tea when suffering from gastroesophageal reflux disease (GERD), as it can make symptoms worse.
- **Baking soda** in warm water can be drunk every 2 hours, but no more than 7 doses.
- Eating too fast can cause indigestion, so sipping **water** throughout the meal will slow you down and soothe any burning.
- Add 2 teaspoons of **caraway** seeds to 2 cups of boiled water, then allow it to steep for 10–15 minutes.

You will need to see a doctor if you are suffering symptoms like excess fatigue, trouble swallowing, unintended weight loss, black stool, vomiting, or appetite loss for longer than two weeks. If indigestion and reflux result in vomiting blood, persistent vomiting, chest pain, or trouble swallowing, see your doctor immediately.

Irritable Bowel Syndrome

Irritable bowel syndrome (IBS) is a digestive disorder that has no cure, and the few available treatments are aimed at treating the symptoms. People with IBS tend to suffer a range of digestive discomforts that range from constipation, diarrhea, bloating, pain, and gas.

Remedies

Those who suffer from IBS tend to have fewer symptoms once they can identify and eliminate foods from their diet that worsen symptoms. Most often, the fewer gas-forming foods you have in your diet, the fewer issues you will have. The low FODMAP (fermentable oligosaccharides, disaccharides, monosaccharides, and polyols) diet works well for a lot of people. However, this isn't a cure, and there are still symptoms. To help cope with those symptoms, try some of the following remedies.

- Many teas that help address digestive issues can be used to alleviate the symptoms of IBS. Sip on teas that include **ginger**, **peppermint**, **slippery elm**, **magnolia bark**, **fennel**, or **chamomile**. **Green tea** may also help with some of the symptoms but can cause bloat in some people. **Berry leaf** teas can help with IBS and high occurrences of diarrhea. **Apple cider vinegar** can also be drunk.

- Consuming **ginger** or **artichoke** in your diet is beneficial. Alternatively, try some **artichoke leaf** bitters or drink some **aloe vera** juice.

- **Milk thistle**, a common weed, can not only help alleviate IBS symptoms but also increase breast milk production. Crush a teaspoon of seeds and add them to a cup of boiled water. Allow the seeds to steep for 5–15 minutes, and drink strained 30 minutes before a meal.

An over-the-counter herbal remedy that can also assist is Iberogast, also known as STW-5. This herbal formulation can be purchased in capsule form.

Continue to eat high-fiber meals, concentrating on those that are magnesium-rich, with the addition of pre and probiotics. However, for some people, high fiber can set off their symptoms, so you will need to monitor what you eat and how it affects you. Lowering stress, getting exercise, and doing some yoga will be beneficial. It's also important to be careful when using laxatives with IBS, as the effects may have unforeseen consequences.

If you notice IBS symptoms are steadily getting worse, with no improvement within 4–6 weeks, then a visit to your doctor is in order. If the problem persists, you may need to see a gastroenterologist.

Nausea and Vomiting

Nausea is a unique feeling that warns you that you're about to vomit. While not all nausea is accompanied by vomiting, it is a debilitating feeling that makes it difficult to concentrate on anything else. Nausea and vomiting can occur for a variety of reasons that range from motion sickness, migraines, eating contaminated food, inner ear issues, and even hunger. If nausea persists it can result in vomiting as the stomach contracts to empty its contents.

Vomiting can be acute or chronic. Acute vomiting is usually sudden and severe, running its course within 2 days. Acute vomiting is associated with motion sickness, pancreatitis, meningitis, food poisoning, excess alcohol, poisoning, and more.

More persistent vomiting is considered chronic and is generally associated with migraines, pregnancy, food allergies, certain medications, and high doses of vitamins due to abusing supplements.

Remedies

While vomiting is a natural survival mechanism, no one enjoys it happening, and even nausea can be debilitating, especially when no clear reason for it occurring can be established. Luckily, there are many ways to deal with nausea and vomiting.

- **Ginger** is considered the panacea for treating nausea. It can be enjoyed as tea or chewed as candied or fresh ginger.
- Another great herbal remedy often used for nausea is **peppermint**. Like ginger, this can be enjoyed as a tea, chewing on the leaves, or sucking on peppermint-containing sweets.
- Many teas that aid in treating gastrointestinal issues can also relieve nausea. Try a cup of **fennel**, **cinnamon**, **turmeric**, **sweet basil**, **cardamom**, or **chamomile tea**.

- Aromatherapy assists in dealing with nausea quickly, and there are various scents that you can choose from. Sniff essential oils such as **ginger**, **peppermint**, **lemon**, **lavender**, **quince**, **orange**, **clove**, **chamomile**, **fennel**, **rose**, and **cardamom**.

- The inclusion of a pinch of **asafoetida** in warm water or foods, such as curry, may help reduce feeling nauseous.

- **Cumin** tea can be made with a tablespoon of cumin leaves or a teaspoon of cumin seeds. Add to a cup of boiled water and allow it to steep for 10 minutes. Don't consume more than 2–3 cups a day.

- **Anise** tea, not to be confused with star anise, is made with a teaspoon of dried, crushed seeds in a cup of boiled water. Cover the cup and allow it to steep for 10 minutes. Drink up to 3 cups a day for only 2 weeks.

- **Clove** tea can also be beneficial. Take up to 10 cloves or a teaspoon and add it to a saucepan with a cup of water. Bring the mixture to a boil, and boil for 5 minutes. Remove from heat and allow it to steep until cool. Drink this up to twice a day.

- While not for everyone, a teaspoon of **onion** juice is said to abate nausea. If the taste and smell put you off, combine it with a teaspoon of freshly grated ginger.

- Rice water is generally something that is thrown away while rinsing rice, but it is a great way to reduce nausea and improve hydration. Take 1/2 a cup of uncooked rice and steep it in 2–3 cups of water for 30 minutes. Strain the rice out, and proceed to simmer the rice water until reduced by a third or half. Drink while still warm.

There are even alternative techniques that can be used to ease nausea and vomiting. Acupressure is one method that is often used to deal with motion sickness. Measure 2 finger-widths distance from your inner wrist and press down firmly with your opposing hand's thumb. You add pressure for a minute and then release it, or you can massage this area firmly for a minute.

Alternatively, try deep breath exercises. Take three seconds to breathe in deeply, hold for three seconds, release the air over three seconds, and hold for another three seconds before starting the next round of breathing.

When drinking different teas or water, take small sips to not irritate your stomach more than it already is. Eating bananas can also be beneficial as the magnesium and potassium present help reduce nausea and deal with any dehydration associated with vomiting.

It's time to seek out a doctor if there is blood in the vomit, a chance of poisoning, dehydration is extreme, there's a lot of pain when vomiting, or vomiting for more than 24 hours. If you find you have a stiff neck accompanying vomiting and a painful head, you must get to a doctor as quickly as possible.

Improving Gut Health

Gut health is vital to your continued health. Due to the length of the gastrointestinal tract, 70–80% of the immune cells in the body can be found around it (Wiertsema et al., 2021). What affects the gut will eventually affect the body's ability to defend itself against anything.

Another aspect to consider when talking about gut health is the gut microbiome, which is filled with trillions of beneficial microorganisms that assist in many tasks that help the body to function at its peak. When the gut microbiome is disturbed due to medication, illness, and poor diet, it finds itself in dysbiosis, allowing pathogenic microorganisms to take over, making you ill.

Remedies

Once the gut doesn't function, the immune system dips and nutrients are poorly absorbed. When the body isn't getting the nutrients it needs and its defenses are down, this is when you can become very ill for extended periods. While many dietary changes can assist in improving gut health, several remedies can also be of assistance, especially if dysbiosis causes digestive issues.

- Consuming fresh **ginger** provides not only fiber but can also assist with a range of digestive issues. It can also be drunk as a tea along with other herbal teas, such as **slippery elm**, **peppermint**, **turmeric**, **cinnamon**, **licorice**, **rosemary**, **cumin**, **cayenne**, **cardamom**, **fennel**, and **cloves**.

- It's also a good idea to improve your diet by cooking with different herbs and spices, such as **oregano**, **rosemary**, **cayenne**, **cumin**, **cloves**, and **fennel**. This will also help reduce your dependency on salt.

The gut microbiome specifically needs nondigestible fiber (prebiotics) as they ferment this to have food. Onion and garlic are great examples to add to your diet. Prebiotics can be found in a variety of fruits and vegetables. Combine this with probiotics to bring new, healthy beneficial microorganisms to the gut microbiome.

Your gut is also affected by stress and low activity. Improving sleep, diet, and getting more active will help your gut to remain healthy. A healthy gut is one with a powerful immune system and an area that can absorb the necessary nutrients to fuel the body.

If you notice worsening symptoms of all other gastrointestinal issues previously discussed occurring, it's time to see a doctor. This is especially true if you're been on heavy antibiotics, as they can cause dysbiosis.

While the gastrointestinal tract is the longest set of organs in the body, that doesn't make it the most important part of the body. However, if unhealthy, it will proceed to drag all other parts of the body down with it. In the next chapter, we'll look at various remedies that can assist with respiratory issues, another vital aspect of our overall well-being.

Chapter 10: Respiratory Remedies

The respiratory system connects your nose and mouth to your lungs, where oxygen is absorbed and carbon dioxide is expelled. When healthy, there is no impact on your breathing.

However, the moment something is amiss, the first signs are usually within the respiratory tract. Whether a tickle in the back of your throat, sudden sneezes, or coughs, these symptoms could be a warning of something worse to come.

Asthma

Asthma is a chronic lung disease that varies from mild to severe. There is no cure, but the symptoms can be managed. Asthma is associated with airway narrowing, and this event may be combined with extra mucus production, making it more difficult to draw breath.

When someone has severe asthma, they must carry a special medication to ensure that airways can be opened quickly to allow enough time to get to an emergency room.

Common symptoms associated with asthma include wheezing, coughing (especially at night or when cold), chest tightness, and shortness of breath.

What triggers an asthma attack is unique to a specific person, so if a trigger can be identified, it's best to avoid it.

Remedies

Due to the inflammation that occurs with an asthma attack, that is what must be targeted to prevent airways from closing. A strong immune system will also assist in reducing symptoms, as this allows the body to fight the triggers more readily. Try some of the remedies below to help lower inflammation and bolster the immune system.

- Try some **ginseng** tea; the recipe is in Chapter 8.
- Other teas you can consider include **turmeric**, **garlic**, and **ginger**. Inhaling the fumes of turmeric tea or its essential oil will also help to open your airways.
- You can include **garlic** (up to 2 cloves a day) and **honey** in your diet. Honey is perfect for treating a cough, as a teaspoon is enough to coat the throat and soothe it.
- **Black seed** oil or powder can be used to help reduce inflammation. While the oil dosage is 0.035–0.088 ounces, you can have 0.035–0.07 ounces of the powder. A professional should determine a more specific dose to deal with a specific condition.
- **Caffeine,** in the form of **coffee** and **regular tea**, is a great addition to the diet as it acts as a bronchodilator, opening airways.

There are even some alternative practices that can assist when suffering asthma symptoms. Determine triggers and eliminate them, try breathing exercises, reduce stress, yoga, and light exercise. However, some people have exercise-induced asthma and should be careful with the types of exercise they do and always carry their inhaler with them.

Asthma can quickly become deadly, so if you find that even after dosing yourself with your inhaler, you're still struggling to breathe, your lips and nails are turning blue, or the skin around your throat and ribs is getting sucked in, you should immediately seek medical attention.

Colds and Flu

Colds and flu are caused by viruses, meaning that antibiotics meant to combat bacteria will do nothing to reduce the symptoms or make you feel better. Colds and flu have similar symptoms, including coughing, sneezing, fever, chills, body aches, and, in some cases, nausea and vomiting. Colds will generally last a week and have lighter symptoms than flu, which can last upwards of 2 weeks.

Remedies

With no medical treatment, at best, some remedies and medications can help alleviate the symptoms and reduce the duration of the diseases. Many of the remedies below will assist in reducing inflammation, fighting pathogenic microorganisms, and simply making you feel better by bringing comfort.

- **Echinacea** has long been used to reduce the symptoms of colds and flu. Take a tablespoon of dried (or 2 tablespoons fresh) echinacea leaves or root and add it to 10 ounces of boiled water. Allow the mixture to steep for 5–10 minutes. The addition of honey or lemon comes with various benefits. An echinacea tincture can also be taken. Consume 30 drops every 3 hours for up to 2 days.

- Eat many different-colored fruits and vegetables. Not only do they contain different antioxidants, but they also contain vitamin C, an antioxidant that improves the immune system. Don't forget to flavor with basil and black pepper, as these can help reduce phlegm.

- Some teas that can help include **ginger**, **lemongrass**, **slippery elm**, **licorice root**, **sweet basil**, **garlic**, **astragalus**, **valerian**, **elderberry**, **cinnamon**, **turmeric**, **clove**, **chamomile**, **lemon balm**, and **peppermint** or **spearmint**. You can even add a few fresh **lemon leaves** steeped in a cup of water to make a lemony tea. You can even keep hydrated and reduce symptoms by enjoying green or black tea.

    - Ginger tea can also be gargled to treat a painful throat.

- **Sage** can be used as a tea or a gargle. Take a teaspoon of dried leaves (or 2 teaspoons fresh) and steep it for 10 minutes in a cup of hot water.

- **Thyme** has powerful antimicrobial properties and can be used in a tea or honey form. For the tea, take a tablespoon of fresh (or a teaspoon of dried) leaves and add them to a cup of boiled water. Steep the mixture covered for 10–20 minutes before drinking hot. For the honey, take 1/2 cup fresh leaves (or 1/4 cup dried) leaves and add them to a saucepan with a cup of honey. Infuse over a low heat for 15–20 minutes, remove from the heat, and allow to cool before straining. Take a teaspoon of the mixture up to 3 times a day.

- For a light, cold-busting tea, take a 5-inch spring of oregano and steep it in 1–2 cups of boiled water for 3 minutes. Enjoy with a teaspoon of honey.

- Create a **yarrow** tea by adding a teaspoon of dried leaves (or 2 teaspoons fresh) to a cup of boiled water. Allow the mixture to steep for 10–20 minutes. This tea should be sipped slowly while still warm. Don't have more than 3 cups per day.

- **Hyssop** tea can be used as an inhalation at the same time. Take a tablespoon of dried hyssop and add it to a cup of boiled water. Allow the tea to steep covered for at least 10 minutes. Season with lemon or honey before drinking it hot while breathing in the steam.

- If you're lucky enough to have **cowslip** growing in your garden, don't poison it. It's great for reducing symptoms of colds and flu. Add an ounce of the dried root to a cup of water in a saucepan. Bring the mixture to a boil before allowing it to simmer for 20 minutes. It's best to avoid if you're on anticoagulants or aspirin.

- **Horehound** (specifically *Marrubium vulgare*) can be used to make syrup to soothe coughs. Take an ounce of dried leaves and add to a saucepan with 2 cups water. Boil for 10 minutes before straining. Measure the liquid and add in double the volume of honey. Mix well and store in the fridge for up to 2 months. Take a teaspoon 4 times a day.

- **Marshmallow** tea is not only naturally sweet but soothes a sore throat and reduces the severity and length of a cough. Take an ounce of dried root and add it to a cup of water before simmering the mixture for 20 minutes.

- Pick 1–2 teaspoons of fresh **mullein** leaves and add them to a cup of boiled water. Allow the leaves to steep for 10 minutes, and then strain well through a coffee filter to get rid of all the irritating hairs.

- **Red clover** can be a pain in the garden, but it's great for colds and flu. Take 1–2 teaspoons of dried flowers and add it to a cup of boiled water, steeping for at least 10 minutes.

- Essential oils in the bath or inhaled over a bowl are a great way to open sinuses that are blocked due to excess mucus. There are many to choose from, so select from **tea tree**, **thyme**, **peppermint**, **marjoram**, **eucalyptus**, **frankincense**, **cinnamon**, **geranium**, **lemon**, and **oregano**. You can even create unique blends to match your taste. If applying essential oils under the nose, add to a carrier oil first. Adding these essential oils to a diffuser could help control pathogenic microorganisms in the air.

- Another way to use inhalations is by adding them to the bath water. Take a cup of dried **rosemary** and add it to 2 quarts of freshly boiled water. Allow it to steep for 10 minutes before straining the liquid and pouring it into your bath water or a foot bath.

- There are over-the-counter salves that can assist in clearing the chest and airways. You can also make your own containing the essential oils of **camphor**, **menthol** (peppermint), or **eucalyptus**. Camphor can be quite powerful and shouldn't be used on children under 2.

- To soothe the throat, take a teaspoon of honey. This will also help reduce coughing. Honey can also be combined with a range of other herbs and spices to help reduce symptoms.
    - Sprinkle some ground **ginger** and ground **pepper** into a teaspoon of **honey** before swallowing the mixture.
- If you have a sore throat, gargle a teaspoon of salt dissolved in warm water.
- **Catnip** is more than an herb to keep your cat happy. By steeping 1–2 teaspoons of dry leaves for 15–20 minutes in boiling water, you create a tea that alleviates symptoms and allows you to sleep better.
- Add 1/4–1/2 teaspoon of **cayenne** pepper in a pint of tomato juice and then drink 1/2–1 cup. The heat from the cayenne will help reduce congestion.
- **Horseradish** can be grated and added to some vinegar to make a dressing for salads that helps soothe the throat. Avoid this remedy if you have issues with your kidneys and gastrointestinal tract.

Unique Remedies

The following remedies are those from around the world. They may not suit your particular tastes but can assist with ailments such as colds and flu.

- Take a small jar, stuff it with chopped **shallots,** and cover them with honey. Stir to combine everything, and top up to keep shallots under the honey. Allow it to steep for up to 2 weeks. Take a tablespoon of the mixture 3–4 times a day.

- **Passion fruit** and **onion** tea can be made by scooping out the inside of 2 passion fruits and combining it with a finely chopped medium onion and 4 cups of water. Allow the mixture to boil for 10 minutes before straining and sweetening with some honey before drinking.

While taking these herbal remedies, it's ideal you remain home and take it easy. After all, rehydration and rest are the best medicines. You can even try some chicken soup, adding a variety of antimicrobial and anti-inflammatory herbs to help fight the infection from the inside.

Another benefit of staying home is that you don't strain yourself or infect others.

If your fever spikes to 100.4 °F, you have trouble breathing, symptoms last longer than 1–2 weeks, you have severe coughing or chest pain, or you produce bloody mucus, it's time to see the doctor.

Congestion

Congestion, otherwise known as a stuffy nose, is sinus pressure caused by the sinus cavities becoming blocked by excess mucus that doesn't drain. This makes it difficult to breathe (especially when sleeping), as well as causes fatigue, post-nasal drip, facial pain, burning eyes, and headaches.

Remedies

Illness, allergies, a deviated septum or nasal polyp, sinusitis, infection, or asthma can cause congestion. While only surgery can help with a nasal polyp or a deviated septum, the rest can be dealt with by removing allergens and using the following remedies to alleviate the symptoms.

- Many warm teas help to loosen mucus and get it draining to reduce pressure. Try drinking teas containing **ginger**, **cayenne**, **peppermint**, **turmeric**, and **black pepper**.

- Essential oils can be used in salves or as inhalations to reduce pressure in the sinus cavities. Try using **camphor**, **eucalyptus**, **oregano**, **rosemary**, **grapefruit**, **peppermint**, or **lavender**.

- **Apple cider vinegar** can be used in a variety of ways. It can be inhaled straight from the bottle, or you can add 2 teaspoons to a cup of warm water and drink that 3 times a day. If the taste puts you off, add up to a tablespoon of honey.

- Honey contains antimicrobial properties, and you can enjoy a teaspoon of it in all your warm drinks, or you can add 2 tablespoons to a cup of lukewarm water to drink.

    - You can also mix a tablespoon of ground black pepper with a tablespoon of honey and add it to a cup of hot water to get both remedies' benefits.

Some alternative therapies you can consider include inhaling steam, using saline nasal spray, using nasal flush with a neti pot, drinking more water, trying chicken noodle soup, using air purifiers, and even a humidifier. You can even apply pressure on either side of your nostrils. Hold for about a minute and release. A warm compress that covers the lower forehead and the upper nose can also assist in getting the mucus to water down. Sometimes, sleeping in a slightly elevated position will assist in draining the sinuses instead of allowing the pressure to build.

Reach out to a doctor if congestion results in a high fever, severe pain, difficulty breathing, chest pain, mucus that is green or yellow, or there is no relief from congestion after 10 days of home treatment.

Coughs

A cough is a reflex where air is forced out of the lungs to clear an obstruction from the airways. It can also occur if there is something that irritates the airways or throat. There are several types of coughs. This includes nocturnal, dry, wet, acute, subacute, and chronic coughs.

Remedies

Coughs are generally caused by allergies, colds, flu, asthma, post-nasal drip, dry air, acid reflux, and to relieve choking. While in some cases, it's to remove an obstruction, in the case of a dry cough, where no mucus is produced, continual coughing becomes tiring and can cause a sore throat. Stop an annoying cough in its tracks with the following remedies.

- **Honey** is the number one remedy when it comes to coughs. All you need is a tablespoon of honey as-is, or you can mix it into warm water or other warm drinks. There are many ways to use honey, such as those outlined below:
    - Take 1/4 teaspoon of **cayenne pepper** and mix it with a tablespoon of honey before dissolving it in a cup of warm water. Drink this mixture up to 3 times a day.
    - Mix a teaspoon of ground black pepper and mix with 2 tablespoons of honey before steeping in hot water for 10–15 minutes. Drink 1–2 cups of the mixture per day.
    - Juice half a **lemon** and add 1–2 tablespoons of honey. Mix well and take a teaspoon when coughing. Alternatively, take a tablespoon of honey to 1/2 teaspoon of lemon juice and mix it into a cup of warm water. Drink this before going to bed.
    - Bake a medium onion until it's soft and blend it with 3 tablespoons of honey. Add a few drops of water to make it more liquid. Take a teaspoon of the liquid up to 3 times a day until coughing starts to improve. Alternatively, juice the onion and drink it with some honey.
    - Add a teaspoon of ground ginger to a tablespoon of honey, and take several times a day to soothe a cough. An alternative to this is using a pinch of cinnamon. Ensure the honey is warm when mixing, but take it cooled. Take 2–3 times a day.

- Another honey blend you can try requires a cup of honey with 3 tablespoons of freshly grated ginger, a tablespoon of dried peppermint, and 4 cups of water. Add the water, ginger, and peppermint to a saucepan and boil the mixture until the mixture is reduced by half. Strain the mixture and add the honey while it is still warm. Take a tablespoon every 3–4 hours. The mixture will last 3 weeks in the fridge.

- Another syrup you can consider is a tablespoon of baking soda mixed into 1/2 a cup of maple syrup. After mixing well, use a tablespoon of the mixture to soothe an irritated throat. You can also try the elderberry and fenugreek syrups below.

- Gargle **salt water** or apple **cider vinegar** for 30 seconds. Mix 2 tablespoons into a cup of warm water. Gargle 1-2 times a day.

- Drink teas that contain **turmeric**, **licorice root**, **thyme**, **ginger**, **peppermint**, **chamomile**, **marshmallow root**, **oregano**, **hibiscus**, **sweet basil** (or chew a few leaves 2–3 times a day), and **lemongrass**.

- If you have access to a guava tree, you can make tea from its leaves. Take 2–3 fresh leaves and add them to a saucepan with a cup of water. Bring the mixture to a boil for 5 minutes. Drink warm once a day.

- You can also try essential oils, such as **thyme**, **eucalyptus**, **peppermint**, **tea tree**, or **thieves oil** (a combination of **clove**, **rosemary**, **eucalyptus**, **lemon**, and **cinnamon**).

- **Carrot juice** soothes the throat and provides all the nutrients needed while fighting illness. Juice 3 large carrots and dilute with water until a cup is filled. Add a few drops of honey and consume up to 3 glasses a day.

- Mix a cup of **pineapple juice** with a pinch of salt and pepper, and 1/2 a tablespoon of honey and store in the fridge, using 1/4 cup up to 3 times a day.
- A teaspoon of honey can also be mixed into a cup of **grape juice** and enjoyed once a day.
- If you can find **jaggery**, all you need to do is put a piece in your mouth and suck on it to help soothe an irritated throat.
- If you are not allergic, take 7–8 almonds, then grind them into a powder before adding them to a glass of orange juice. Sip this juice.

Recipes

Try some of the following recipes to make your own cough syrups.

Elderberry Cough Syrup (Kukreja, 2023)
Ingredients

- 3 1/2 c water
- 1/2 tsp cloves
- 1 c raw honey
- 2 tbsp fresh ginger root, grated
- 1 tsp cinnamon powder
- 2–3 c dried black elderberries

Directions

1. Keeping the honey aside, add everything to a saucepan and bring it to a simmer.

2. Simmer for 30–40 minutes or until the volume is reduced by half.

3. Remove from heat and use a potato masher to crush the berries.

4. Set aside and allow the mixture to cool, then strain.

5. Once completely cooled, pour in the honey and mix well.

6. Keep the syrup in the fridge and take a tablespoon to ease a cough. Take up to 3–4 times daily until symptoms improve.

Fenugreek Cough Syrup (Kukreja, 2023)
Ingredients

- 2 c warm water
- juice of one lemon
- 2 tbsp fenugreek seeds
- 3 tsp dried thyme
- 1 c of honey
- 3 cloves
- 3 tsp dried oregano
- 5 tbsp extra virgin olive oil

Directions

1. Grind the seeds into a powder.
2. Pour the warm water into a bowl and add the oregano, seed powder, thyme, and cloves. Set aside covered for 15 minutes.
3. In a saucepan, add the olive oil with the honey, and keep the heat low. Stir the mixture until the honey and oil are fully incorporated.
4. Strain the infusion and add it to the saucepan. Keep the temperature low and continue to mix until everything is well combined.
5. Pour in the lemon as you stir, then remove the saucepan from the heat.
6. Let the mixture cool before you bottle it.
7. Take a tablespoon of the mixture 3–4 times a day.

See your doctor if the coughing produces blood, there's a high fever, chest pain, or shortness of breath.

Hay Fever

Hay fever, also known as allergic rhinitis, is an allergic reaction to grass and pollen. It usually peaks during spring but can occur throughout the year. This is a seasonal allergy that doesn't affect everyone, but if it affects you, it can make spring a miserable time of year.

Remedies

Hay fever causes an itchy nose, watery eyes, congestion, sneezing, coughing, headaches, excess mucus, nausea, post-nasal drip, and blurred vision in severe cases. In some cases, medication works well to control symptoms; in others, give the following remedies a try.

- If you're not allergic to honey, you can try micro-dosing yourself with **honey** or **bee pollen** to help you build up a resistance to pollen-related allergies. Ideally, get locally so you can become resistant to local flora.
- Consider adding adaptogens to your diet, as they can help the body adapt to the stress of the season. Add food such as **ginseng**, **reishi mushrooms**, **tulsi**, **chaga mushrooms**, **maca**, **ashwagandha**, **garlic**, **onion**, and **water hyssop**.
- Some teas that can help include **elderberry**, **turmeric**, **chamomile**, and **licorice root**. You can even enjoy some **aloe vera juice**.
    - If you have **elderberry** syrup, dose yourself 1–2 teaspoons a day.
- Take a cup of fresh **stinging nettle** leaves and add them to 2 cups of boiled water. Allow them to steep for 5 minutes before straining through a coffee filter to reduce the chance of irritating hairs. Serve with some honey or lemon.
- Some essential oils that could assist include **chamomile**, **eucalyptus**, and **frankincense**.

    - A chamomile inhalation can be made with 4 tea bags in a large bowl with hot water. Drape a towel over your head and breathe in the steam.

Hay fever can generally be treated at home. However, if the symptoms last longer than four weeks and you have been experiencing them for at least four days, it may be time to talk to your doctor.

Sore Throat

Pharyngitis, or a sore throat, can be caused by various problems such as viral or bacterial infections, allergies, upper respiratory tract infections, smoking, sleeping with an open mouth, or even severe coughing.

Remedies

A sore throat is annoying and debilitating. While throat lozenges can offer temporary relief, they never last long enough. The following remedies help soothe the inflammation and fight back against any pathogenic microorganisms causing the infection.

- Two of the most common remedies for sore throat are combining **lemon**, **ginger**, and **honey** or a **hot toddy**.
    - Add the juice of half a lemon and combine it with 1/2 cup of hot water, a teaspoon of honey, and a

teaspoon of ground ginger (or a 1/2-inch piece of fresh ginger, grated). Steep everything together for 5 minutes, and drink it still warm, straining if necessary.

  - For a hot toddy, you'll need a tablespoon of lemon juice, an ounce of whiskey, a tablespoon of honey, and enough warm water to fill a cup. Stir and drink warm before going to bed.

- Cut a **garlic** clove in half and place a piece in each cheek and suck for a few minutes. Alternatively, chew the clove.

- Gargle **salt water** for 5–7 minutes up to 2–3 times daily.

- Create a **baking soda** gargle by adding 1/2 teaspoon of salt and 1/2 teaspoon of baking soda and mixing it in a cup of warm water. Gargle for a minute up to 3 times daily.

- Try some teas that contain **sage**, **chamomile**, **licorice root**, **slippery elm**, **marshmallow**, **peppermint**, **fenugreek**, **cayenne**, **echinacea**, **ginger**, and **cinnamon**.

  - Teas such as sage can also be gargled.

- When using steam, try adding a few drops of **eucalyptus**.

  - If you can find food-grade **peppermint oil**, add a few drops to an ounce of plant-based oil to create a throat spray.

- Chew on a few **cloves**, but remember to rinse your mouth afterward to remove the numbing sensation.

- **Apple cider vinegar** with some honey and lemon in warm water will help soothe your throat. Alternatively, sipping **lemon water** will offer relief.
- A tablespoon of **honey** helps heal and soothe a burning throat. Alternatively, try up to 2 tablespoons of **coconut oil** in a warm beverage daily to help lubricate mucus membranes.

Alternative therapies include using steam, drinking more to increase hydration levels, and using an air humidifier. Even soups and broths will help you feel better.

Recipe

Throat sprays offer targeted relief from a burning throat. Sage and echinacea both offer soothing and healing properties to a sore throat.

Sage-Echinacea Throat Spray (Spritzler, 2024)
Ingredients:

- 1/2 c boiled water
- 1 tsp ground sage
- 1 tsp ground echinacea
- 1/2 c vodka

Directions:

1. Add the sage and echinacea to the boiling water and allow it to steep for 30 minutes.

2. Strain the liquid and pour the vodka into the mixture.
3. Decant the mixture into a spray bottle.
4. Use the spray every 2 hours until pain subsides.

Generally, sore throats heal by themselves, but in some cases, it can be a sign of something worse. See a doctor if your tonsils are swollen enough to reduce breathing while sleeping, there's severe pain, a fever over 101 °F for more than 2 days, the sore throat lasts longer than a week, or a red rash starts to spread.

Sinusitis and Allergies

Allergies can be caused by many things ranging from pollen to pet dander. Allergies can cause sinusitis as well as watery and burning eyes, sneezing, runny or blocked nose, feeling ill, clogged ears, and facial pain.

Remedies

You can treat allergies and sinusitis the same as hay fever. However, allergic reactions can get worse over time, so it's important to identify what is causing the reaction so you can deal with it before anaphylaxis can occur.

- As with hay fever, a spoonful of **honey** could assist in building up resistance to allergens.

- In the case of congestion, there are many essential oils you can use, such as **eucalyptus**, **sandalwood**, **frankincense**, **rosemary**, **ravensara** (not safe for use on children), and **lavender**.
- You can also use teas that contain **butterbur**, **stinging nettle**, **peppermint**, **spearmint**, and **ginger**.
- Try a small glass of **pineapple juice**. Pineapple contains bromelain, which decreases swelling and improves breathing.

Alternative therapies include nasal irrigation, increasing vitamin C intake, consuming more probiotics, and acupuncture.

The biggest issue that could arise from allergies is anaphylaxis, a severe allergic reaction. This can cause chest pain, trouble swallowing or breathing, heart palpitations, wheezing when trying to breathe, hives, vomiting, dizziness, and abdominal pain. If anaphylaxis occurs. If anaphylaxis occurs, you'll need an EpiPen and a trip to the emergency room. -- To keep it active and possibly make it a little smoother.

With so many remedies to treat respiratory problems, you're spoiled for choice and can stick to your favorites. However, there may be many other ways to combine remedies. I encourage you to keep researching to find those that best suit you. In the next chapter, we'll concentrate on remedies that deal with the urinary tract.

Chapter 11: Bladder Remedies

The urinary system or urinary tract removes waste and excess fluid from the bloodstream. The system consists of two kidneys connected to two ureters, which lead to the bladder, sending urine through the urethra and out of the body. Anatomically, those born with female-presenting genitalia are likely to develop more problems with their urinary tract than those born with male-presenting genitalia. Below are some of the ailments that could affect the urinary tract.

Urinary Incontinence

Urinary incontinence, also known as an overactive bladder or leaking bladder, is an embarrassing and potentially dangerous condition that can lead to infections that can affect the urinary tract. This ailment can be caused due to aging, diabetes, and even an enlarged prostate, but that doesn't mean it can't be corrected.

Remedies

Urinary incontinence can be identified as either wet or dry. A dry, overactive bladder will leave you with the urge to urinate, but nothing happens when you try to urinate. A wet, overactive bladder is when there is leakage before you can make it to the bathroom, as the bladder muscles are contracting strongly with you having no control. You may even find that you get up several times a night to relieve yourself, disturbing sleep. Here are a few remedies that may assist with the problem.

- Improve your diet by adding magnesium-rich foods, such as cashews, kale, pumpkin, and bananas, as these foods improve the health of your kidneys.
- There are a variety of teas you can try, but do so 1–2 hours before going to bed. Try teas containing **cayenne**, **horsetail** (Chapter 7), **mullein**, and **green tea**.
- **Gosha-jinki-gan** (GJG) is a traditional Chinese remedy that blends 10 herbs that assist with many bladder issues. This is available over the counter, and each product will have a dosage you should observe.
- **Saw palmetto** tea is particularly good for those with an enlarged prostate. Add 1/4 cup of fresh berries (or 2 tablespoons of dried berries) to 2 cups of boiling water. Cover and allow the mixture to steep for 15 minutes. It can be flavored with 1/4 teaspoon of vanilla essence and a tablespoon of honey. The berries strained from the mixture can be used to make a second batch.
- **Bladderwrack**, a type of seaweed, can be used as a tea to reduce symptoms. Take a teaspoon of dried bladderwrack and add it to a cup of water before simmering the mixture for 10–15 minutes.
    - This remedy is high in iodine, and you shouldn't drink more than 2 cups of it a day. Avoid using this remedy if you have an overactive thyroid, use any other remedies that contain iodine, or take hormones for hypothyroidism.

- **Corn silk**, the corn beard, is often used by Native Americans to treat bladder issues. Take the corn silk from 3–4 corn ears and trim the ends before allowing them to dry overnight. Add these to 3 cups of hot water and steep for 5 minutes.

- **Reishi**, also known as lingzhi, mushrooms can also be used. Take 1/4 ounce dried mushroom and add it to 8 cups of water in a saucepan. Allow the mixture to boil before reducing it to a simmer for 30–60 minutes. The longer you simmer, the stronger the tea. Allow to fully cool before drinking. Some ginger can be added during the simmering step to improve the taste if you wish.

- Take a tablespoon of dried **buchu** leaves and add them to 2 cups of boiled water. Let the mixture steep for 5–10 minutes. The longer you steep, the more bitter the drink. This tea can also be combined with chamomile or peppermint to assist with sleep.

- A teaspoon of **crataeva** bark can be steeped in a cup of boiled water for 10–20 minutes. Drink 1–2 cups daily.

Urinary incontinence isn't caused by a single problem, but thankfully, there are many ways to deal with it. Some changes you can make include getting rid of alcohol, reducing inflammatory foods, reducing smoking, lowering weight, and avoiding drinking too close to bedtime.

There are even some exercises you can do to train your bladder. There are even some exercises you can do to train your bladder, such as Kegel exercises. These help strengthen the pelvic floor, allowing you to hold urine longer. Alternatively, you can exercise bladder control, and when you feel the urge to go, you hold for 5–15 minutes to strengthen all the muscles involved.

Ideally, you should go to your doctor as soon as you notice strange and concerning changes to the frequency or urgency of urination. Ignoring bladder issues for too long can cause infections that can travel up to the kidneys.

Bladder Infections

Commonly known as bladder infections, urinary tract infections (UTIs) can occur anywhere along the urinary tract and are most commonly caused by the bacteria *E. coli*. The infection is most often associated with a burning sensation when urinating, increased intensity or frequency of urination, discolored or bloody urine, fatigue, and fever. It can also be accompanied by pain in the lower abdomen, back, or pelvis.

Remedies

A bladder infection shouldn't be allowed to continue for too long without treatment, as the damage can become irreversible. In most cases, the infection can resolve itself through the use of antibiotics or several herbal remedies, as outlined below.

- To your diet, add apples, oranges, and cranberries. These fruits contain **D-mannose**, which could assist in preventing pathogenic bacteria from attaching to the cells in the urinary tract, making it easier to flush them out.
- Teas not only help with the symptoms of bladder infections but also hydrate you, so more liquid and possible bacteria

are flushed out of the urinary tract. Try teas such as **green tea**, **ashwagandha**, **cranberry**, **parsle**y (from Chapter 7, but don't add the essential oils), **chamomile**, **peppermint**, **corn silk**, **horsetail**, and **hibiscus**.

- **Bearberry leaf** tea is a powerful remedy that should only be used at the onset of bladder infection. Take 0.1 ounces of dried leaves, and add it to 6.5 ounces (roughly a teacup) of cold water. Allow the mixture to infuse in a cool, dark area for 12–14 hours. Drink a teacup full up to 4 times a day, and don't continue for longer than a week.

- **Juniper berries** can also help, but be careful which you use, as some species have poisonous berries. Only use the berries from *Juniperus communis*, *J. drupacea*, and *J. phoenicea*. Add a teaspoon of dried juniper berries to a cup of boiled water and allow it to steep for 10–15 minutes. Add honey or lemon to taste. Avoid using this remedy if you have kidney disease.

- **Goldenseal** can be used as a tea or tincture. When taking the tincture, use 0.01–0.035 ounces 3 times a day. For the tea, mix 2 teaspoons of dried leaves or a teaspoon of root powder into a cup of hot water. Allow the mixture to steep for 10–15 minutes, and drink 2–3 times daily.

- Not to be confused with goldenseal, **goldenrod** tea can also assist in fighting bladder infections. Add 2 tablespoons of the dried leaves to a cup of boiled water, allowing the leaves to steep for 10 minutes. Drink a cup of this tea several times a day.

- **Dandelion** tea contains vitamin C and many other compounds that can treat bladder ailments. Take 0.5 ounces of fresh leaves or roots and add them to a cup of boiled water, then steep for 5–10 minutes. Drink 2–3 times a day.

- **Boxwood** tea can be made by adding 1–2 teaspoons of dried leaves to a cup of boiled water. Steep for 5–10 minutes before drinking. Drink up to 3 times a day.

- Take a teaspoon of dried **wild radish leaves** and steep them in a cup of boiled water for 5 minutes. Enjoy 2–3 cups daily.

- **Garlic** is antibacterial, so consume more of it. You can also combine garlic with ginger to make a unique tea. Cut 3 cloves of garlic is half and add them to the saucepan with 3 cups of water. Bring it to a boil. Once boiled, remove from the heat and add 1/2 teaspoon ground ginger and honey to taste. Allow the mixture to steep for 5 minutes before straining and drinking.

- If you have access to **giloy** (heart-leaved moonseed), you can crush a 12-inch stem piece with a pestle and mortar. Add the crushed giloy to a blender and add 2 cups of water. Blend for a few minutes before straining, and drink a cup in the morning and a cup in the evening.

- **Pomegranate juice** can also be enjoyed. However, this remedy may interact with medications that lower cholesterol. Take the seeds from 2–3 ripe pomegranates and add them to a blender with a cup of water. Blend for a few minutes before straining and drinking.

- In the recipe section below, you can find the instructions to make a **nasturtium tincture**. Take 20–50 drops in 1/2 cup of water 3–5 times daily.

Recipe

Nasturtium Tincture (Adamant, 2023)
Ingredients:

- nasturtium flowers, fresh or dried
- vodka

Directions:

1. Fill a mason jar with the flowers and cover with vodka.
2. Stir to cover all the flowers, keeping them below the alcohol level.
3. Seal the jar and shake before adding it to a cool, dry location for 6–8 weeks.
4. Every few days, give the jar a gentle shake.
5. If the alcohol level drops, add more.
6. At the end of extraction, strain the tincture through cheesecloth and transfer it to a new, amber-colored container.
7. Label and store for later use.

Mild UTIs usually resolve themselves, but sometimes, the infection from the bladder can travel up into the kidneys. This results in a high fever, chills, diarrhea, back pain, nausea, and vomiting. Once this occurs, speak to your doctor to culture your urine and get treated with antibiotics.

Kidney Stones

Kidney stones develop for many reasons, such as not adequately hydrating or having excess salts or minerals (such as oxalates, calcium, and uric acid) in the diet. In many cases, these stones are small enough to pass from the kidneys out of the body without you even knowing they exist. However, when these stones get too big, they can be painful to pass and, in severe cases, may need medical intervention to get rid of them.

Remedies

Ideally, you want to prevent the development of kidney stones by watching what you eat. However, everyone is unique, and there is a chance that you may be more prone to developing kidney stones than others. Here are a few remedies that can help prevent the creation of stones and, in some cases, help partially dissolve them, making them easier to pass.

- Drink **water**, at least 8 glasses a day. The exact number you may need will depend on your activity level, age, and gender. Ideally, you want to produce pale yellow urine with little to no smell to indicate your hydration levels.

- Add half a cup of **lemon** juice to 1/2 a cup of water. Use fresh lemon juice, not reconstituted juice, without diluting it appropriately. Increasing acidity helps dissolve stones.

- To a cup of warm water add 2 oz of **olive oil**, 2 ounces of **lemon juice**, and 2 ounces of **apple cider vinegar**. Mix well and drink up to twice a day.

- There are many teas you can try, such as **sweet basil**, **dandelion**, **stinging nettle**, **hibiscus**, **parsley**, **horsetail**, and **bearberry**.
    - **Basil** can also be enjoyed in meals or infused in water. Alternatively, crush enough leaves to fill a teaspoon and mix it with a teaspoon of honey. Enjoy up to 3 times daily.
- **Java** tea, not to be confused with coffee, can be made with 0.21 ounces of dried leaves steeped for 10–15 minutes in 4 cups of boiled water. Enjoy 2–3 times daily.
- **Chanca-piedra** (gale of the wind or stonebreaker) tea has long been used to treat kidney stones. To 4 cups of boiled water, add 0.7 ounces of chanca-piedra dried leaves and steep for 15 minutes. Drink a cup up to 3 times a day.
- **Florida burhead tea** (also known as miner's tea) can be made with 0.7 ounces of dried leaves added to 4 cups of water. Boil the mixture for 10 minutes before straining and allowing to cool. Drink 2–3 cups daily.
- To make **black mulberry leaf** tea, take 0.53 ounces of dried leaves and add it to 4 cups of boiled water. Allow the leaves to steep for 15 minutes and drink up to 4 times daily.
- Try the juice of **pomegranate**, **celery**, or **wheatgrass**. For celery juice, take 1–2 celery stalks and blend until mostly liquid. Strain and top up with water. Apples can also be juiced with the celery. Wheatgrass can similarly be juiced. However, this is a potent herb, and it's best to only drink small volumes at a time.
- While it may seem counterintuitive, add 1/2 teaspoon of **baking soda** with 2 tablespoons of **apple cider vinegar**.

Allow the mixture to mix before consuming it. This remedy can be taken twice a day. Alternatively, add 1/4 teaspoon of baking soda to a large spoonful of honey before mixing into a cup of water and drinking it.

Large kidney stones that can't be passed cause internal damage as they travel through the urinary tract. This results in chills, fevers, bloody urine, severe pain, nausea, and vomiting. Depending on the size of the stone, treatment can vary from medication to ultrasonic energy or surgery. Reviewing your diet and decreasing alcohol consumption would be helpful. Eating foods such as kidney beans and olive oil will improve health and reduce the risk of kidney stones.

When you first notice changes in your urine, including its frequency, it's a good idea to ask yourself what you have been doing that day or the day before. Most urinary problems stem from not hydrating correctly and can be fixed by improving your water intake along with some electrolytes. If this doesn't help, try a few remedies before reaching out to your doctor.

Now, let's leave the internal organs for a while to look at the very organ that prevents us from dehydrating to death: the skin.

Chapter 12: Skin Remedies

Your skin is the largest organ of the body. It serves as a physical barrier that maintains moisture, helps thermoregulate, and prevents germs and chemicals from entering your body. The skin has its own microbiome, like your gut, that needs to be looked after. It's also a sensory organ that reacts to temperature, pressure, and moisture changes. It's the first line of defense for your body. It's crucial to protect it and keep it healthy. Alas, it, too, can be affected by many different ailments, but thankfully many treatments can help.

Psoriasis

Psoriasis is an autoimmune disease that causes excess skin to be created, making the affected areas scaly, swollen, red, and itchy. While this is annoying, the skin can also crack, creating entry to a range of bacterial, fungal, and viral infections.

Remedies

Psoriasis is a chronic condition, and as of yet, there is no cure. However, there are many ways to deal with the symptoms and prevent possible secondary infections. Below, you can find soothing remedies and some suggestions to prevent further irritation of the affected skin.

- One of the best remedies is taking a soothing, warm bath. Combine this with **oatmeal** (Chapter 6) or **Epsom salts**. Take 1–2 cups of Epsom salts, dissolve it in a warm bath, and soak for up to 20 minutes. You can alternatively use Dead Sea salt.
    - You can also add 2 teaspoons of olive oil to your bath.
- **Turmeric** tea can be drunk or applied to the skin as a warm compress.
- A **chamomile** infusion using 4 tablespoons of fresh flowers steeped in 2 cups of boiled water for 5–10 minutes, should be allowed to cool completely before using. Pour the mixture over the scales and air dry. Use this treatment 3 times daily.
- Remove the gel from an **aloe vera** leave and make a compress, keeping it in place for 20–30 minutes up to 3 times a day. Continue this treatment for 4 weeks.
- Eat more omega-3 fatty acids to reduce inflammation from many chronic conditions.
- A 1:1 ratio of **apple cider vinegar** to water helps to lower itchiness from the scales.
- Many salves offer relief from the symptoms of psoriasis. Try your hand at making the **Oregan grape salve** below. Not only does it soothe, but it has antibacterial properties.
- A **baking soda poultice** (Chapter 6) or a **calendula poultice** can be applied directly to affected areas. Take 3–4 fresh calendula flowers and mash them with a mortar and

pestle before applying them to the scales. Leave the poultice in place for 15–20 minutes before washing away and then air drying the area. Be wary of a reaction and wash the area thoroughly if this occurs.

- Not only is **watercress** considered a superfood, but it makes an amazing anti-psoriasis tonic. Take 2.5 ounces of fresh watercress and blend it with a cup of water. Drink the tonic up to 3 times a day. Alternatively, incorporate it into your diet.

- Essential oils, such as **tea tree** and **pine bark** can be added to a carrier oil and applied to the affected area. **Olive oil** and **coconut oil** are excellent carrier oils but can also be used as is to help moisturize the skin.

Why psoriasis develops is not fully understood, but what makes it worse is understood. Avoid dry air using a humidifier, reduce stress, and keep the scales moisturized to prevent them from cracking. Steroid creams can be used under the guidance of a doctor. To help your body heal from the inside out, add more fruits and vegetables with beta-carotene (such as those that are yellow and orange) and increase omega-3 fatty acids.

Contact your doctor or dermatologist if your joints start to swell, feel painful or warm, and fail to function as they should. Pain in the lower back may accompany this.

Recipe

The Oregan grape has long been used to treat skin conditions, so try this salve to reduce the symptoms of many different skin conditions.

Oregan Grape Salve (Sierralupe, n.d. -a)

Ingredients:

- 10 drops tea tree essential oil
- 3 oz beeswax, grated
- 2 cups almond oil
- 1/2 dried Oregon grape root
- 4 garlic cloves, chopped
- 10 drops geranium essential oil
- 1/2 cup dried mullein leaf

Directions:

1. Heat the almond oil over the lowest heat in a double boiler.
2. Once warm, add the garlic and Oregan grape root, and then add the lid.
3. Keep the oil warm, but not steaming, for 4–8 hours to infuse the oil.
4. During the last 30 minutes of infusing, add in the mullein leaf.
5. Strain the solids from the oil, returning the oil to the clean double boiler.
6. Add the beeswax and raise the temperature to medium until the wax is melted.

7. Turn the heat off and allow the mixture to cool for a few minutes before adding the essential oils and stirring.
8. Pour the salve into tins and allow to cool until solid.
9. Seal the tin, label it, and store it in a cool, dark place.

Boils and Carbuncles

Boils are pus-filled bumps that can become large and painful over time. As they grow, they form abscesses, and when several boils are clustered together, they're known as carbuncles. All are associated with redness, swelling, pain, and pus, although the pus won't necessarily leak. Boils are caused mostly by the bacteria *Staphylococcus aureus*, which enters the hair follicles or oil glands under the skin. The most affected areas are the eyelids, armpits, buttocks, shoulders, and groin.

Remedies

Boils are easily treated at home. The number one piece of advice all doctors give is that a boil never be popped. Not only can this be painful, but there is also a chance that pus goes into the body (leading to sepsis) or spreads the bacteria that caused the boil in the first place to the rest of your skin. Follow these remedies to reduce a boil.

- The best remedy is to draw out the infection with a **warm compress**. Soak a piece of absorbent cloth with warm water, wringing out most of the liquid, and then add it to the boil for 20 minutes. This can be used 3–4 times daily until the boil disappears.

    - Alternatively, add some **Epsom salts** to the warm water and soak a cloth in the mixture. Use this remedy for 20 minutes up to 3 times a day.

- Essential oils such as **tea tree**, **tridax daisy** (coat buttons), **caraway**, or **eucalyptus** can be added to a carrier oil and then added to a cotton ball to be dabbed onto the boil 2–3 times daily.

- Other topical treatments you can add to the boil include **castor oil** (3 times a day), **neem oil** (3–4 times a day), and **honey**.

    - Create a blend with a teaspoon of vinegar, 1/2 teaspoon of honey, and 1/2 teaspoon of lemon juice, and then add it to the boil. Allow it to air dry for 40 minutes before washing it off. Use this remedy twice a day.

- To help your body fight the infection and inflammation, try teas such as **turmeric** or **ginger**.

- Poultices are a great way to draw out infection. Try using **turmeric** (fresh or dry), **ginger** (fresh or dry), **tridax daisy** (poultice or tincture), **devil's horsewhip** (poultice or tincture), **aloe vera** gel, or **toothpaste**.

    - Take a tablespoon of turmeric powder and mix it with 1/2 a tablespoon of crushed ginger. Create a paste by adding the mixture to some water or coconut oil.

- Add a slice of **onion** or use an **onion tincture** to help reduce the boil and the possibility of scarring. Crushed **garlic** can also work. Crush the garlic, add it to the boil, then place a cool compress over the garlic for 20 minutes. Do this every 12 hours. Garlic may not be suitable for sensitive skin.

- A thin slice of **potato** can be tied to the boil overnight, or you can use potato juice-soaked gauze. Take a small potato and grate it, squeezing all the juice from it. Soak the liquid into a piece of gauze and tie it in place for a few hours. Rinse the area and repeat up to 3–4 times a day.

Using home remedies will help resolve boils in 2-21 days. If there is no sign of improvement while using remedies, the boil continues to grow (as large as a ping pong ball), clusters of boils develop, there's extreme pain, or red streaks develop outwards from the boil (cellulitis), it's time to speak to your doctor.

If you're a diabetic or have a problem with a boil recurring every few months in the same area, it's advised you also speak to your doctor. A doctor should always treat carbuncles as they may need to take a culture to determine what is causing the infection.

In the case of a boil bursting, wash the area thoroughly with antibacterial soap and then cover the wound in sterile gauze. Ensure your hands are clean at the time of treating and changing dressings.

The dressing can be changed every few days, but more frequently if they get dirty. Keep clothing and bedding clean during the healing process to prevent other bacteria from entering the wound.

Eczema

Eczema, otherwise known as atopic dermatitis, is a chronic skin condition that causes inflammation, redness, and itching. Anyone can be affected by eczema. In severe cases, the dry, itchy patches can become swollen with blisters, which can crack open, opening the body for secondary infections from bacteria and fungi.

Remedies

Eczema can be treated at home with home remedies or over-the-counter medications in most cases. Allergies and environmental conditions are generally the cause. So, if you notice dry, damp, or cold weather causes eczema or if you're prone to allergies, you'll need to make a few lifestyle changes. Regardless of what triggered it, several remedies can alleviate the symptoms of eczema.

- **Oatmeal** is one of the gentlest ways to treat eczema. Try the oatmeal cream in the recipes section below, or consider an oatmeal bath and then apply a moisturizer. For babies with eczema, try the anti-eczema baby balm in the recipes section.

- A **cool compress**, with or without oat milk, can reduce itchiness. A **comfrey** compress (Chapter 6) can also be used.

- Topical treatments you can consider include **aloe vera** gel, **coconut oil** (which can be used as a carrier oil as well), **honey**, **calendula** wash (Chapter 6), **chamomile** (use tea bags after the steeping process), **dandelion** salve (recipe below), **milk thistle** tea (Chapter 9), **stinging nettle** (tea or poultice), **St. John's wort** tea (Chapter 8), **turmeric** tea, **sunflower** oil, **witch hazel extract**, **petroleum jelly**, **echinacea** tea, and **ginger** tea.

    - **Milk thistle** tea can also be created with a tablespoon of dried leaves instead of seeds.

    - All teas can be applied as washes or drunk.

- Some helpful essential oils include **tea tree**, **calendula**, **chamomile**, and **dandelion**.

- While not for everyone, diluted **bleach** can assist in killing any bacteria that infect the eczema. Take 1/4–1/2 cup of plain bleach, and add it to a full bathtub. Soak for only 10 minutes, and then rinse yourself with clean water. This remedy should only be done 2–3 times weekly.

Alternative therapies you can consider include switching to sensitive skin hygiene products, eating more anti-inflammatory foods, avoiding dry heat, protecting your skin from cold air, using fabric softeners (or avoiding if allergic), reducing stress, trying acupressure, and not scratching.

In the case of sensitive skin, it may be a good idea to speak to a dermatologist before trying any herbal remedies or OTCs in case there is an underlying condition causing the eczema.

Generally, eczema only requires medical intervention if the itching prevents you from sleeping or doing any other activities, it worsens (even with treatments), infection sets in, there is severe pain, or you get a fever.

Recipes

The following recipes aim to reduce the symptoms of eczema and bring relief from inflammation and itching.

Oatmeal Cream (Pedersen, 2023)
Ingredients:

- 2 tbsp honey
- 10 drops lavender essential oil
- 1/2 c oatmeal, ground finely
- 1/4 c coconut oil

Directions:

1. Add the oatmeal, coconut oil, honey, and lavender oil to a bowl and then stir to combine.
2. Using clean fingers, take some of the cream and rub it into the affected skin, and then leave it in place for a few minutes to be absorbed.
3. Wash the excess cream away with lukewarm water.
4. Dry your skin by gently patting it.
5. Excess cream should be stored in an airtight container in a cool, dry place.

Anti-Eczema Baby Balm (Pedersen, 2023)
Ingredients:

- 2 tbsp coconut oil

- 1 tsp oatmeal, ground finely
- 1/4 c shea butter

Directions:

1. In a double boiler, add the shea butter and coconut oil and melt over medium heat. Stir until well combined.
2. Remove the mixture from the heat and allow it to cool for a few minutes.
3. Sprinkle in the ground oatmeal and stir.
4. Transfer the mixture to a clean, airtight container, and then allow it to solidify.
5. This balm is gentle enough to use on babies with nappy rash.

Eczema Balm (Pedersen, 2023)
Ingredients:

- 10 drops rose hip essential oil
- 1 tbsp cocoa butter
- 1/4 c aloe vera gel, blended smoothly
- 2 tbsp olive oil

Directions:

1. Melt the cocoa butter in a double boiler over medium heat.
2. Once melted, pour in the olive oil, stirring to combine.

3. Remove the mixture from the heat and allow it to cool for a few minutes before adding the aloe vera gel.

4. Stir until everything is well incorporated.

5. Add the essential oil at this stage.

6. Pour the balm into a clean container and allow it to solidify completely.

7. Once solid, seal the container and place it in a cool, dark area until ready to use.

Dandelion Salve (Berry, n.d.)
Ingredients:

- 0.5 oz beeswax pastilles
- 3.5 oz dandelion-infused oil

Directions:

1. In a double boiler, add the oil and beeswax and melt over medium heat. Stir to mix well.

2. Remove the double boiler from heat and add the balm to a clean container.

3. Keep the salve stored in a cool, dark area sealed until ready to use.

Dandruff

Dandruff is identified by an itchy scalp, which produces white flakes of skin. This oftentimes embarrassing condition is caused by being sensitive to certain hair products, a fungal infection caused by *Malassezia* yeast, dry skin, or seborrheic dermatitis.

Remedies

Dandruff generally isn't something you need to bother your doctor with, as there is a range of herbal remedies and anti-dandruff shampoos that can deal with the problem. Here are some of the best remedies you can make at home.

- **Tea tree** oil is most often used for a range of skin conditions. A few drops of the essential oil can be added to your shampoo or in a carrier oil. **Lemon grass** essential oil can be used in the same way.

- Use topical applications such as **coconut oil** (can also be used as a carrier oil), **aloe vera** gel, **olive oil**, or **apple cider vinegar** (1:1 ratio with water and can also be used together with essential oils).

    - To use apple cider vinegar, make up the correct dilution and add it to hair that has already been washed. Allow it to dry for 15 minutes before rinsing it with water. Use this remedy once every 2 days.

    - Add olive oil to the scalp and wash after 10 minutes, or wrap your head in a towel and allow the oil to be absorbed overnight.

- Crush 2 **aspirin** tablets and mix them with the usual volume of shampoo you use to wash your hair. Apply it to the scalp, massage it in, and rinse thoroughly.

- Take a tablespoon of **Listerine** and add it to 9 tablespoons of water before pouring it over the scalp. Wash away with anti-dandruff shampoo to get rid of potential pathogenic microorganisms.

- Combine **coconut oil** and **lemon**. Take 2 tablespoons of coconut oil and add 2 tablespoons of lemon juice. Massage into the scalp and leave in place for 20 minutes before rinsing off with shampoo.
    - Alternatively, add 2 tablespoons of salt to this mixture and make a scrub. Gently massage into the scalp and leave in place for 7–10 minutes before rinsing with shampoo.
- A teaspoon of **fenugreek seeds** can be soaked in water overnight before mashing into a paste. Add a splash of lemon juice before adding to the scalp. Allow the mixture to sit for 30 minutes before washing hair.
- **Neem** paste can be made with a few leaves crushed into a paste. Add to the scalp and allow to rest for 10 minutes before rinsing with water.
- After enjoying an **orange**, take the peel and add it to a blender with a splash of lemon before blending until a paste is formed. Apply the paste to the scalp for 30 minutes before washing away with shampoo. Use this remedy up to 3 times a week.
- Add an **egg yolk** to your scalp and massage it in before adding a plastic bag over the hair. Keep the bag in place for an hour before washing your hair. If the egg smell lingers, wash your hair a second time. This remedy can be done 3 times a week.
- Crush a few **sweet basil** leaves with 2 teaspoons of water and 2 teaspoons of amla powder to make a paste. Add to

scalp and leave to dry for 30 minutes. The paste can be rinsed away with water. This remedy can be used daily and can even strengthen hair.

- Take a medium **banana** and mash it into 2 cups of **apple cider vinegar** to create a paste. Apply the paste to the scalp and massage it into the entire head. Wash with shampoo after 20 minutes.

- Pour some lukewarm **green tea** over your head and allow it to dry for 30 minutes before rinsing with water.

- Crush 2–3 **garlic** cloves with a tablespoon of **honey** and apply it to the scalp. After 15 minutes, rinse with shampoo.

Some lifestyle changes help reduce the symptoms of dandruff. This includes reducing stress, increasing intake of omega-3 fatty acids, consuming probiotics, and reducing foods that could bolster fungal infections (such as refined carbohydrates, processed foods, sugary foods, or fried foods). Increase your intake of fruits, vegetables, vitamin B-complex, and zinc.

If dandruff symptoms don't improve in 2–3 weeks after trying home remedies, or worsen, it's time to turn to your doctor or dermatologist for medical options or further suggestions of home remedies. If you suffer from psoriasis or eczema, speak to your doctor before trying home remedies.

Acne

Acne is annoying, and most people will have it at some point in their lives. It is caused by sebum, a natural oil produced by the skin, that starts to clog pores along with dead skin cells. These blocked pores can then become infected with *Propionibacterium acnes*, which results in cysts and pustules.

Remedies

The inflamed and puss-filled bumps associated with acne are annoying and embarrassing but can easily be treated from home. There are many reasons you could be suffering from acne, ranging from certain medications, smoking, endocrine disorders (such as polycystic ovary syndrome), restrictive clothing, genetics, stress, diet, air quality, poor hydration, and poor sleep are just some causes. Thankfully, many remedies can help.

- Many essential oils and carrier oils can assist with the symptoms of acne. Try **tea tree**, **echinacea**, **rosemary**, **manjistha**, **neem**, **calendula**, and **lavender**. The best carrier oils include **argan oil**, **coconut oil**, and **jojoba oil**.
    - Tea tree oil can be added to water in 1:9 dilution before being applied to treat spots. Can be added to skin 1–2 times daily.
- Some teas that can be drunk or applied to the acne include **green tea** (the tea bags can also be added to the skin), **echinacea**, **chamomile** (use the tea bags as well), **spearmint tea** (made the same way as peppermint tea), **ginger**, **lemongrass**, and **turmeric**. **Amla juice** can also be drunk.
    - **Neem** tea made with 5 fresh or dried leaves or a 1/4 teaspoon of dried bark can be added to a cup of warm

water and left to steep until cool. This tea should be drunk, but the longer the steeping period, the more bitter. Add some honey or reduce the steeping period.

- Create a poultice using a few **chamomile flowers**. A poultice can also be made with **peppermint**. Take 2 tablespoons of chopped fresh peppermint and mix it with 2 tablespoons of finely ground oatmeal and 2 tablespoons of plain yogurt to form a paste. Apply to the face and leave it for 10 minutes before rinsing off with water.

- Other topical applications you can use include **aloe vera** gel, **honey**, **witch hazel** extract, and **toothpaste**.

- **Apple cider vinegar** can reduce symptoms and reduce the appearance of scarring. Mix the vinegar and water to a 1:3 ratio and add it to the skin with a cotton ball. Leave the liquid on the skin for 5–20 seconds before rinsing and patting the skin dry. Apply remedy 1–2 times daily.

- To the juice of a **lemon**, add a few drops of **rose water**, and then use a cotton ball to dab it onto the affected skin.

- Make a face mask using 2 tablespoons of **honey** to a teaspoon of ground **cinnamon** paste. Add it to a clean face and keep it on for 10–15 minutes before rinsing and patting the skin dry.

- A **brewer's yeast** mask is also effective. Combine a packet of brewer's yeast with a tablespoon of lemon juice or water to make a paste. Apply it to a clean face and leave it in place for a few minutes before rinsing off with lukewarm water and patting it dry.

- To help remove dead skin cells, you can make an exfoliate. Create a **sugar** and **coconut oil** paste in a 1:1 ratio and apply it to the skin with a gentle massage before rinsing away with warm water. Do this daily.

Some lifestyle changes you should consider are not touching the affected skin (no popping zits), using the correct cleansers for your skin type, using oil-free facial products, hydrating, getting more exercise, and reducing stress. Diet can play a large role. Improve your diet by eating more fish, seeds, and nuts while reducing dairy and high glycemic index (GI) foods.

See your doctor when the acne covers large areas, creates dark spots, becomes painful, becomes a recurring problem, doesn't respond to home treatments, breakouts continue for years, becomes infected, occurs over thighs or upper arms, causes emotional distress (reduction in self-esteem), and the acne affects the skin deeply. Know what medication you're on, as there is a chance it can cause acne.

Vitiligo

Vitiligo is an autoimmune condition that affects the skin (and occasionally the mucus membranes and hair) that causes the melanin pigment cells to be slowly destroyed. This ailment affects all people but is more readily noticed in those with darker skin. Small white patches first appear before they steadily start to grow.

The cause of the disease is unknown, though some people believe that it may be hereditary or could be caused by diseases that affect the endocrine system or connective tissue. Stress may also play a role.

Remedies

Vitiligo normally affects skin that is exposed to the sun and cannot be cured. While there is no way to know if you'll develop the disease, there are ways to possibly prevent it by helping the body generate melanin cells with the following remedies.

- **Papaya juice** can be drunk, or a piece of the fruit can be rubbed along the white patches. Drinking this remedy helps to boost the body's ability to make new melanin cells.

- Create a **red clay poultice** by mixing 2 tablespoons of clay with a tablespoon of ginger juice and applying it to the patches. The copper content helps to improve melanin production.

- Add enough **turmeric** and **mustard oil** to make a paste, and then add it to the patches. Keep it in place for 20 minutes before washing off. Do this twice a day.

    - Consuming turmeric may cause worsening vitiligo and possibly prevent repigmentation (Wilde, 2021).

- Other poultices you can make include **sweet basil** with some **lemon juice** and fresh **ginger**.

- Some essential oils that could be used include **babchi (bakuchi)**, **bergamot**, **thyme**, **black pepper**, **frankincense**, **lavender**, and **turmeric**. Combine with **coconut oil**, **castor oil**, **black seed oil**, or **neem oil**.

- As **copper** helps with melanin production, drink water from a copper container. **Ginko** tea (Chapter 8) can also be enjoyed. The addition of **black pepper** to food will also be beneficial.

- Eating up to 5 **walnuts** a day will also be beneficial. Alternatively, use **walnut powder** (made from ground-up shells) with some water to create a paste. Add to the patches 3–4 times daily for 15–20 minutes.

Recipe

This unique blend of oils and essential oils seeks to assist in reducing vitiligo while boosting your body's ability to make more melanin.

Vitiligo Essential Oil Blend
Ingredients:

- 3 drops black seed oil
- 3 drops black pepper essential oil
- 3 drops thyme essential oil
- 2 tbsp jojoba oil

Directions:

1. Add all the ingredients in a small glass container. Seal and shake to combine.
2. To use, add a few drops to the affected area and gently massage into the skin.

3. Use the oil 1–2 times daily. Keep the container in a cool, dark place when not in use.

Some lifestyle changes you can make include reducing stress, using sunscreen, and consuming more vitamins B12, B9, and D. It's also a good idea to have your thyroid checked, as vitiligo has been linked to an underactive thyroid (Wilde, 2021). Increasing your iodine intake may assist with this.

If vitiligo develops suddenly, it may be a good idea to talk to your doctor about possible home remedies you'd like to try. In some cases, your doctor may suggest some medications. If the ailment worsens, further steps can be discussed with your doctor or dermatologist, especially if you have other chronic or thyroid conditions.

Looking after your skin has many advantages, as it's the largest organ that protects you from the outside world. You have a better chance of protecting your health as long as it's healthy. Now it's time to return to inside the body to see how to improve your reproductive health.

Chapter 13: Reproductive Health Remedies

Reproductive health is vital as it not only affects the development during puberty but can also have wider effects throughout adulthood. The reproductive organs differ between those assigned female or male at birth, while the hormones are similar. However, the concentrations of these hormones vary between genders as they develop.

Those assigned as female have ovaries, fallopian tubes, a vagina, a cervix, and a uterus and will develop breasts once puberty hormones start to circulate. Those assigned as male at birth have a prostate, a penis, and testes and will develop stronger muscles and bones when puberty hormones start circulating. These genders will undergo many changes during puberty to prepare the body for adulthood.

With so many changes, there is always a chance of something not going as planned, especially as you age. Thankfully, there are ways to deal with ailments that affect sexual health from the comfort of your home.

Erectile Dysfunction

Also known as impotence, erectile dysfunction (E.D.) is the struggle to get or maintain an erection firm enough to have sexual intercourse (Fletcher, 2023b). Most men will likely experience this at least once in their lifetime due to many reasons, such as emotional distress, stress, anxiety, and blood flow issues, to name a few.

Remedies

For an erection to occur, there is a mixture of emotions, hormones, sexual organs, blood flow, muscles, and the nervous system that play a role. If anything disrupts one of these factors, erectile dysfunction can occur. As this ailment can happen for several reasons, several remedies could assist.

- There are several teas you can try. Consider drinking **ginkgo**, **ginseng** (only for 6–8 weeks), **green tea**, **chamomile**, **cinnamon**, and **ajwain**.

- You can create a **powerful spiced tea** by adding an inch of cinnamon, a teaspoon of jeera seeds, 5–7 cloves, a teaspoon of fennel seeds, a teaspoon of coriander seeds, 2 slices of fresh ginger, and a teaspoon of black pepper to a saucepan with 1–2 cups water (depending on the strength preference). Boil the mixture for 5–10 minutes and then steep it a further 10 minutes before straining and drinking.

- Combine the power of **ginseng** with the calming effects of **peppermint**. Add 0.07 ounces of dried ginseng root to a cup of water and boil it for 10 minutes. Remove from the heat, sprinkle in a teaspoon of dried peppermint leaves, and allow it to steep for 5–10 minutes. Add a tablespoon of honey and drink up to 3 cups a day.

- **Yohimbe** tea can be made with a teaspoon of dried bark steeped in boiled water for 30 minutes. Enjoy with a splash of lemon. This tea can be drunk twice a day for no more than 10 days. A high dose can cause an increased heart rate, seizures, heart attacks, and kidney failure. If you're on antidepressants or stimulants, discuss using this remedy with your doctor.

- **Horny goat weed** has long been touted as an effective remedy for E.D. in China. Supplements can be bought over the counter, or you can make tea. Place a teaspoon of the dried week in a saucepan with a cup of water before boiling it for 10–15 minutes. Drink once cooled.
- To make **catuaba** tea, use 0.09 ounces of the bark and add it to a cup of water before boiling for 15 minutes. Remove the mixture from the heat and allow it to cool. Drink up to a cup a day.
- **White's ginger** (*Mondia whitei*) is a remedy from Uganda that helps improve libido and low sperm count. Add a teaspoon of powdered root to a cup of hot water and allow it to steep for 5–10 minutes. Strain and sweeten before drinking.
- **Marapuama** tea can be made with 2 tablespoons of bark and added to 4 cups of water before boiling together for 15 minutes. Drink up to 3 cups a day, but avoid if you have heart issues or high blood pressure.
- Place a whole **nutmeg** in a cup of boiled tea and allow it to steep for 15 minutes before drinking.
- **Maca**, also known as Peruvian ginseng, helps to reduce stress and E.D., particularly the black maca. Take 0.1 ounces a day in a smoothie or juice. However, it's best to avoid it if you have a heart condition, as maca can increase blood pressure.

    - Make a watermelon-maca juice by adding 3 large slices of watermelon (fruit only) and 3 teaspoons of maca powder to a blender. Split the drink into 3 servings and drink throughout the day.

- Any essential oil that can reduce stress should assist with E.D. Try sniffing **lemon** to help improve mood.

- A commonly used supplement that can be purchased is **L-arginine**. The dosage will be determined by the product and brand purchased.

Many E.D. problems stem from a poor lifestyle, and it only takes a few changes to start improving your sex life once more. Try getting some light exercise along with improving your diet, weight, cholesterol, and blood pressure. It will also assist if you reduce alcohol consumption, stop smoking, reduce stress, and try alternative therapies such as yoga and acupuncture.

Speak to your doctor if E.D. occurs regularly or if it starts to affect your life. Erectile dysfunction could be a sign of underlying conditions, such as diabetes, heart disease, and blood pressure problems, so a physical may be in your best interest. Some treatments could include medications (such as Viagra), therapies, and possibly surgery.

Menstrual Cramps

The menstrual cycle is the build-up of the uterine lining (made of endometrial cells) to welcome a fertilized egg at the start of pregnancy. However, the egg isn't always fertilized, and the lining cannot remain forever. To get rid of this blood-rich lining, the uterus contracts powerfully, resulting in the lining being lost through the vagina. This causes a period that can last 2–7 days and occurs on average every 28 days but can vary from 23–35 days in length.

This cycle affects all those with uteruses from the time of puberty to menopause, roughly once a month. In many cases, the menstrual cycle is somewhat painful, lasting a day or so, and then there is little to no pain later, but this isn't true for everyone.

Remedies

The cramps are caused by the uterus to be rid of the uterine lining. For some, the pain can be debilitating, starting at the beginning of the period and lasting several days. The pain is usually at its worst during the first few days before easing toward the latter days.

The pain is normally situated in the lower abdomen but can also affect the lower back, upper thighs, and groin. The following remedies seek to ease the cramps and make your period slightly less miserable.

- **Heat** is your best friend, as it relaxes your muscles. Soak in a bath or add a hot water bottle to the area with the most pain.

- Abdomen massages will greatly assist with the pain. This can be combined with a range of essential oils, such as **peppermint**, **clary sage**, **Roman chamomile**, **rosemary**, **fennel**, **turmeric**, **rose**, **pine bark**, **dill**, and **lavender**. Warm the carrier oil before adding the essential oils for maximum effectiveness.

- Try teas that contain **berry leaf** (especially **red raspberry**), **dandelion**, **chamomile**, **fennel**, **ginger**, **licorice root**, **cinnamon**, **angelica root** (Chapter 9), **peppermint**, **oregano**, **green tea**, and **basil**.

- **Lavender** can help calm and reduce pain, so try it as a tea. Take an ounce of dried leaves, and add it to 4 cups of boiled water. Steep the mixture until cool and drink up to 3 times a day. Avoid this tea if you have gastric ulcers.

- If you want a hint of spring, try the **marigold mix** tea. Take a small handful of fresh marigold flowers, a teaspoon of fennel seeds, and a teaspoon of ground nutmeg and place it in a saucepan with a cup of water. Boil together for 10 minutes. Drink this remedy up to twice a day.

- **Mango leaf** tea can be drunk up to 2 days before your cycle starts to help lower pain. Take 0.7 ounces of dried leaf and boil it with 4 cups of water for 5 minutes. Drink up to 4 cups a day with a teaspoon of honey.

- **Wormwood** tea with some honey will be bitter but helpful. Add a tablespoon of fresh leaves to a cup of boiled water and steep for 5 minutes. Drink 2-3 cups daily. Avoid this remedy if breastfeeding.

- Traditional Chinese medicine likes to combine **licorice root**, **cinnamon**, **angelica**, and **red peony root** when making menstrual cramp medication. The dosage of these mixtures will vary between practitioners.

    - A **red peony root** decoction can be made by adding a tablespoon of dried root to a cup of water and allowing it to simmer for 20 minutes. A low simmer is a must; don't boil the water.

- **Chasteberry**, also known as Vitex, tea can be made with a teaspoon of dried flowers and 10 ounces of water. Allow the 2 to boil together for 3–4 minutes, then set aside to steep for 10 minutes. Drink up to 2 cups a day for no longer than 3 months. This remedy should only be used by those 18 or older. A high dose can result in intestinal issues.

- **Pycnogenol**, made from pine bark extract, is an OTC that can be taken during the period to help relieve pain.

- A **dill supplement**, up to 1,000 mg daily, can be taken up to 2 days before your cycle to reduce pain.

Recipes

If you want something a little stronger than just a single essential oil to relieve your pain, try the following recipes to help relieve period cramps.

Anti-Cramp Salve (Marie, 2015)
Ingredients:

- 4 drops German chamomile essential oil

- 0.67 oz safflower oil (or carrier oil of choice)

- 6 drops juniper essential oil

- 40 drops clary sage essential oil

- 30 drops peppermint essential oil

- 20 drops cassia essential oil

- 20 drops chili seed essential oil
- 6 drops lavender essential oil
- 0.25 oz beeswax

Directions:

- Melt the beeswax into the safflower oil in a double boiler.
- Once well combined, remove from the heat and allow the mixture to cool for a few minutes.
- Add the various essential oils and stir.
- Pour the still liquid salve into a waiting tin and allow it to cool completely before storing.
- To use, apply the salve to your abdomen when the cramps start and leave it on for 5–10 minutes to allow the warming effect to start.

Period Pain-Relief Salve (Tekurio, 2023)
Ingredients:

For infused oil

- 1 cup avocado oil (or carrier oil of choice)
- 1 part lavender flowers
- 1 part white willow bark
- 1 part helichrysum flowers
- 1 part chamomile flowers

For salve

- 1 cup infused oil
- 8 drops sweet marjoram essential oil
- 8 drops juniper berry essential oil
- 8 drops clove essential oil
- 8 drops lavender essential oil
- 2 tbsp beeswax

Directions:

1. Add enough herbs for the oil infusion to allow the oil to cover them. Add a little extra oil if required. However, you will only be using a cup of infused oil for the rest of the recipe.

2. Store the container in a cool, dark area for 4–6 weeks. Alternatively, use the heat method to get a quicker oil infusion.

3. Strain the herbs from the oil and retain a cup of the infused oil.

4. Add the beeswax and infused oil to a double boiler and heat over medium until the wax is fully melted. Stir to combine.

5. Allow the mixture to cool for a few minutes before adding the essential oils. Stir well.

6. Transfer to containers to cool and solidify before sealing and putting away.

7. To use, rub along the lower abdomen or back when the cramping begins.

Some alternatives you can try include gentle exercise (such as stretching or walking), yoga (including poses such as cobra, clank, child, and cat-cow), having an orgasm (helps the uterus contract and then relax), or acupuncture.

Dietary changes that could help include eating more omega-3 fatty acids, hydrating more, and consuming more fiber while reducing the consumption of poor fats, alcohol, and caffeine.

While many people who have menstrual cramps reach for OTC pain relief, when you're suffering from extreme pain, heavy bleeding, cramps worsen as you get older, or the cramps interfere with your daily life, it's time to reach out to your doctor. There is a chance that underlying conditions, such as endometriosis or polycystic ovary syndrome, can cause the extreme pain.

Endometriosis

Endometriosis is a chronic and painful condition where the endometrial tissues that normally grow within the uterus start to grow outside of it. These cells can attach to the fallopian tubes, the outside of the uterus, ovaries, and any tissues that attach to the uterus. These cells react to the menstrual cycle, causing severe pain, heavy bleeding, nausea, as well as localized pain in the pelvis and back.

Other symptoms that can occur include possible bleeding between cycles, pain when urinating or having bowel movements, pain during intercourse, fatigue, and digestive issues.

The cause of endometriosis is mostly unknown, though hormonal imbalance, genetics, and environmental factors may play a role. Endometriosis isn't curable and can affect fertility and cause cysts.

Remedies

Endometriosis can affect 10–15% of those with uteruses (WebMD Editorial Contributors, n.d.-a). Many who suffer the ailment often resort to pain management, hormonal drugs, and even surgery to get relief from extreme and extended pain.

Thankfully, there are a few remedies that can assist.

- Many teas can help with the inflammation and pain associated with endometriosis. Try teas that contain **turmeric**, **chamomile**, **peppermint**, **chasteberry**, **ashwagandha**, **ginger**, **motherwort** (Chapter 8), **green tea**, and **rosemary**.
- **Pycnogenol** can be used with oral conceptions to help reduce the symptoms of endometriosis.
- Similar to menstrual cramps, certain essential oils in a warm carrier oil can be massaged into the abdomen to reduce pain. Try using oils such as **pine bark**, **lavender**, **rose**, **clove**, and **cinnamon**.
- Add **flax seeds** to your salads, as the omega-3 fatty acids help reduce inflammation.

Recipes

Try the following recipes to reduce inflammation and pain caused by endometriosis.

Ginger and Turmeric Tea (*Three Recipes to Help Ease*, n.d.)
Ingredients:

- 1–1 1/2-in fresh turmeric, peeled
- 1–1 1/2-in fresh ginger, peeled
- 1 pineapple, peeled and chopped
- 1–2 whole lemons, cut into quarters
- a dash of extra virgin olive oil

Directions:

1. Add everything to a juicer or blender and process until smooth.
2. If using a blender, strain the mixture and retain the liquid.
3. Drink a small shot glassful every 1–2 hours until the pain abates.

Red Raspberry Jellies (*Three Recipes to Help Ease*, n.d.)
Ingredients:

- 1 cup strong raspberry leaf tea (Chapter 9, double the number of leaves but keep water volume the same)
- agar flakes

- 2 cups raspberries, fresh or defrosted (any berries can be used)
- 1 1/2-in fresh ginger, peeled and grated

Directions:

1. Add the tea, ginger, and raspberries to a blender and process until smooth.
2. Strain the mixture through cheesecloth over a measuring cup. Take note of the volume.
3. Pour the liquid into a saucepan and add a rounded tablespoon of agar flakes per cup of liquid.
4. Raise the temperature to obtain a simmer, not stirring. Don't allow the mixture to boil.
5. Once simmering, stir occasionally as the agar flakes dissolve over 3–5 minutes.
6. Transfer the liquid to jelly molds or ramekins.
7. Leave the molds to cool to room temperature before transferring to the fridge.
8. Help yourself up to 1/4 of the jelly a day, more if the symptoms are at their worst.

A change in diet may reduce the symptoms. Increase your omega-3 fatty acids and antioxidants, and add anti-inflammatory foods to your diet. Avoid consuming trans fats, and reduce sugar and processed foods. Exercise will release endorphins, making it easier to deal with the pain.

If your periods become too painful, you bleed too heavily, or you have spotting throughout your cycle, it's time to talk to your doctor about what could be causing your endometriosis.

Polycystic Ovary Syndrome (PCOS)

PCOS, also known as Stein-Leventhal syndrome, is a common endocrine condition that can't be cured but can be managed. This ailment affects 7% of those assigned as female at birth (Barode, 2024c). The causes of this ailment are still not fully understood, but hormone issues and insulin are the most common explanations, while genetics may also play a role.

Common symptoms associated with PCOS include but aren't limited to unwanted hair growth, thinning scalp hair, increased weight, possible infertility, ovarian cysts, acne, and irregular periods.

Remedies

While many treatments can reduce the symptoms associated with PCOS, it's a one-size-doesn't-fit-all situation. It may be in your best interest to speak to your doctor before trying herbal remedies to have their assistance in choosing which may be best for you, especially if you are on other medications or herbal remedies. Below are some of the remedies that could help.

- Many teas can help reduce inflammation and balance

sugar. Try teas that contain **cinnamon**, **turmeric**, **ashwagandha**, **holy basil**, **licorice root**, **chasteberry**, **black cohosh** (Chapter 8, the tincture can also be used), **flaxseed**, **chamomile**, **fenugreek**, **fennel**, **ginger**, **peony**, **spearmint**, **St. John's wort**, and **dandelion**.

- **Evening primrose** is high in omega-3 fatty acids, which can help reduce inflammation. Supplements are purchased over the counter, or you can make a tea. Take 1–2 teaspoons of dried flowers or leaves and steep them for 10 minutes in a cup of boiled water. Avoid this remedy if on anticoagulants or phenothiazines. Evening primrose can have serious side effects in high doses, such as reduced blood clotting, nausea, diarrhea, and inflammation.

- Other supplements that can be considered for the diet include omega-3 fatty acids, vitamin D combined with C, vitamin B-complex, chromium, selenium, and inositol. Maca root, flax seeds, and saffron can also be added to meals. Try adding the maca root to aloe vera juice.

- ***Tribulus terrestris*** (**goathead** or **devil's thorn**) can help ovulation and possibly reduce ovarian cysts. Take a teaspoon of the dried herb and steep it for 5–7 minutes in a cup of boiled water.

- ***Dong quai***, also known as female ginseng, is a tea made from a tablespoon of dried root boiled with 2 cups of water for 15–20 minutes. Drink it warm after straining and adding lemon or honey.

- Make **marjoram** tea by adding 1/4 teaspoon of the dried herb to a cup of boiled water. Allow the herb to steep for 3 minutes, and drink with a teaspoon of honey.

- Take a heaped teaspoon of dried **shatavari** root and steep it in a cup of boiled water for 5–10 minutes. This tea pairs well with peppermint or lemongrass.
- Essential oils you apply or sniff include **tea tree** and **lavender**.

Recipes

Enjoy the following PCOS remedies to soothe the most annoying symptoms.

Sugar-Balancing PCOS Tea (*Herbal Tea*, 2019)
Ingredients:

- 1 tsp fenugreek seeds
- 1/2-inch ginger crushed
- 3 c water
- 1 handful peppermint leaves
- 1-in cinnamon stick
- 1/2 tsp licorice root powder
- 2 stalks of lemongrass
- 8–10 basil leaves
- 2 tsp honey or sweetener of choice (optional)

Directions:

1. Add all the ingredients to a saucepan and bring it to a boil.
2. Continue boiling until water is reduced by a third.
3. Strain and add optional honey.
4. Enjoy hot or cold.

Nourishing Morning Tea (Gupta, n.d.)
Ingredients:

- 1 tsp lemon juice
- 1/2-inch cinnamon stick
- 1 teaspoon fennel seeds
- 1/2-inch fresh ginger piece
- 5–6 fresh peppermint leaves
- 1 c water

Directions:

1. Boil a cup of water in a saucepan and add the herbs and spices.
2. Cover, then lower the temperature to a simmer.
3. Simmer the mixture for 5–10 minutes.
4. Steep and serve with the lemon.

Spiced PCOS Infusion (Purwar, 2023)
Ingredients:

- 2 cups water
- 1 tsp fennel seeds
- 1 tsp coriander seeds
- 1 tsp crushed cumin seeds
- 1 tsp crushed cardamom
- 1 tsp dry rose petals

Directions:

1. Add all the ingredients to a bowl, cover, and steep for at least 3 hours in the fridge.
2. Strain and enjoy.

A nourishing, anti-inflammatory diet is often suggested to help reduce insulin resistance and help with PCOS. Aim for whole foods rich in iron (especially protein), magnesium, vitamins, and probiotics. Avoid or reduce sugar, refined carbohydrates, and caffeine (which may cause changes in hormonal levels).

Other beneficial lifestyle changes include maintaining a healthy weight, doing low-impact exercise (high intensity could worsen symptoms), reducing sleep, improving sleep hygiene, and getting acupuncture.

It's a good idea to remain in contact with your doctor, as those with PCOS are at risk of developing uterine cancer, type 2 diabetes, heart disease, and high blood pressure.

Menopause

Menopause is when the estrogen level starts to drop in those assigned as female at birth. This is something that will eventually happen, usually at around 50 years old. Menopause occurs when you haven't had a period in a year. Before menopause occurs, you may have irregular periods until they eventually stop completely. Symptoms that occur during menopause include vaginal dryness, insomnia, night sweats, hot flashes, depression, a reduction in bone density, and more. These symptoms can last 5–10 years.

Remedies

Menopause is annoying and can be debilitating, often resulting in people turning to hormone therapy to reduce the symptoms. However, this isn't without its own risks. While an age-related ailment, there is no reason to suffer it. Not when many home remedies can ease the symptoms.

- Many teas that assist with PCOS symptoms can also assist with menopause. Try teas that include **evening primrose**, **black cohosh**, **angelica root**, **ginseng** (works well with sleep disturbances), **St. John's wort**, **flaxseed**, **red clover** (Chapter 10), ***dong quai***, **kava kava**, **valerian** (tea and tincture), and **chasteberry**.
    - Many herbal remedies contain plant hormones that can mimic estrogen.
    - Warm drinks drunk during hot flashes can worsen the symptoms. If this occurs, enjoy your tea cold.

- Try adding **maca powder**, **flaxseeds**, or **flaxseed oil** to your diet, as having an anti-inflammatory diet will reduce symptoms.

Some lifestyle changes you can consider include meditation, exercise, reducing hot drinks, reducing alcohol consumption, and maintaining a healthy body weight.

Seek out a doctor's assistance if the symptoms are unmanageable or you suddenly start period-like bleeding after not having a cycle in over a year. There is a correlation between severe hot flashes and night sweats and an increased risk of cardiovascular disease, so be sure to tell your doctor about them.

The most important part of reproductive health is not being afraid to talk about it. Never ignore problems, as there is likely always an underlying issue, or they could worsen. With that in mind, let's look at ailments that affect musculoskeletal structures.

Chapter 14: Musculoskeletal Remedies

We have all overdone training or have experienced a fall. Besides some abrasions, these injuries normally affect joints and muscles, causing sprains, strains, and sore joints. Sometimes, you don't even need to do something to injure yourself, and old injuries can flare up later in life.

Aches and pains slow you down and make it difficult to enjoy your life. While some people can work through the pain, it's generally not advisable, as aches and pains are the body's way of telling you something is wrong. However, pain is subjective, as one person's 10 could be another's niggling discomfort. Regardless, it's a good idea to deal with the underlying problem causing the pain.

Joints (Arthritis)

The most common discomfort to joints, excluding injury, is arthritis. Arthritis is the swelling of the joints. These joints will be painful, inflamed, stiff, have reduced movement, and may even be red. Common arthritis types include rheumatoid arthritis and osteoarthritis. Your diet can play a role in joint issues as well. In my case, once I removed gluten from my diet, my severe back pain became more manageable. While I wasn't gluten-intolerant, I was sensitive, and this led to inflammation and pain.

Remedies

Joint pain is mostly caused by repetitive motion and injury, age, and obesity. While there isn't much you can do about injuries that have occurred in the past, there is plenty you can do with the painful symptoms that are happening at this moment. Below, you'll find remedies that assist in reducing inflammation and pain.

- Topical treatments such as **aloe vera** gel, essential oils (including **eucalyptus**, **borage seed**, and **chili seed**), and salves that include **devil's claw** (recipe below), **thunder god vine**, and **cat's claw** can all assist in pain and inflammation management.
    - **Arnica-infused oil** is particularly good for pain, whether from joint pain or bruises. Add a cup of dried flowers to a saucepan with 3 cups of olive oil. Allow the mixture to simmer for 4 hours. Monitor the temperature closely and stir every 30 minutes. Strain the flowers from the oil and store them for later use. Apply the oil as is or use it in other salves.

- Try teas that contain **boswellia** (Chapter 8, 0.035 ounces is enough), **ginger**, **green tea**, **turmeric**, **willow bark** (Chapter 8), **cinnamon**, **ginkgo**, **stinging nettle**, **thyme**, and **aswagandha**.

- **Thunder god vine** is well known for treating joint pain, but when taking supplements, it's best to talk to a naturopathic physician to get the correct dosage and formulation. Creating a home extract can result in deadly consequences if made with the incorrect parts.

- Spices that will improve inflammation and can readily be added to your food include **garlic**, **black pepper**, and **cayenne pepper**.
- **Evening primrose** oil, roughly 0.089 ounces, can be taken daily but can take up to 6 months to show results.

Recipes

Joint pain doesn't have to make your life miserable; try some of the following remedies to ease the pain and inflammation.

Devil's Claw Salve (Stewart, n.d.)
Ingredients:

- 1 tbsp beeswax
- 1 tsp cocoa butter
- 6 tbsp devil's claw-infused oil (made with the root)

Directions:

1. Add all ingredients to a double boiler over medium heat until the wax is melted. Mix well.
2. Pour the salve into a prepared container and allow it to cool and solidify.
3. Apply to painful joints as needed.

Anti-Arthritis Tea (*Recipe: Soothing Osteoarthritis Tea*, n.d.)

Ingredients:

- juice of a small lemon
- 10 oz boiled water
- 1 1/4-in fresh ginger piece, grated
- pinch cayenne pepper
- 1 tsp ground turmeric
- 1 tsp honey or sweetener of choice
- pinch ground pepper

Directions:

1. Add all the spices to the boiled water and stir it for 2–3 minutes.
2. Stir in the honey and leave the tea to steep until it reaches your preferred temperature.
3. Strain and pour in the lemon juice.

Anti-Inflammatory Tincture (*Turmeric Black Pepper Tincture*, n.d.)

Ingredients:

- 1 c vodka
- 1/4 c water
- 1 tbsp whole black peppercorns

- 1/4 lb fresh turmeric, washed and diced in a food processor

Directions:

1. Add all the ingredients in a jar and set it aside for 2–4 weeks to infuse.
2. Gently shake the container every few days. Add extra vodka if required.
3. Strain the solids and transfer the tincture to an amber-colored container.
4. Use 20–30 drops 2–3 times daily.

Joint-Soothing Salve Recipe (*Joint Pain Salve*, n.d.)
Ingredients:

- 10 drops ginger essential oil
- 6 drops rosemary essential oil
- 10 drops peppermint essential oil
- 12 drops turmeric essential oil
- 10 drops eucalyptus essential oil
- 10 drops pine essential oil
- 7 drops helichrysum essential oil
- 15 drops lavender essential oil
- 0.8 oz beeswax pellets
- 3.2 oz unrefined coconut oil

Directions:

1. Mix all the essential oils in a glass container.

2. Melt the beeswax in a double boiler over medium heat and add the coconut oil. Mix until the oil and wax is well combined.

3. Remove the mixture from the heat and allow it to cool for a few minutes.

4. Pour in the essential oils and stir until well incorporated.

5. Decant the salve into a container and allow it to solidify over 24 hours.

6. Gently rub into inflamed joints as needed.

Joint-Soothing Ointment (Axe, 2023)
Ingredients:

- 20–30 drops myrrh essential oil
- 10 drops pure ginger essential oil
- 20–30 drops frankincense essential oil
- 4 oz unrefined coconut oil, warmed to be liquid

Directions:

1. Add the essential oil to the liquid coconut oil and stir until well combined.

2. Transfer the ointment to a clean container and store it in a cool, dry place.

3. Massage into painful areas twice a day.

You can even make some lifestyle changes to improve joint pain. Try losing some weight, decreasing stress, using hot and cold treatments, light exercise (especially stretching and yoga), and getting a massage. Meditation may also assist in dealing with the pain while waiting for the remedies to kick in. Because rheumatoid arthritis is a chronic condition, an anti-inflammatory diet is necessary.

Joint pain is something many people live with. However, if you find the pain is severe, the joint isn't usable, the shape seems off, or if the swelling doesn't abate after three days (even with intervention), it's time to seek out a doctor. An underlying condition may cause joint pain.

Sore Muscles

An injury or overuse can cause joint pain and sore muscles. It's generally a warning from the body that you should relax and take the time to heal. However, that doesn't mean you need to sit in pain while recovering.

Remedies

For muscle soreness or stiffness, the main treatments are pain management and reducing inflammation. Unless there is a blatant injury that requires a doctor or hospital visit, sore muscles can be treated from the comfort of your home. Here are a few remedies you can use.

- Use essential oils, such as **lavender**, **rosemary**, **wintergreen**, **chamomile**, **peppermint**, **eucalyptus**, **lemongrass**, and **marjoram**.

- Anti-inflammatory and pain relief teas include those made with **turmeric**, **tulsi**, **fennel**, **ginger**, **cloves**, **cinnamon**, **lemongrass**, **green tea**, **stinging nettle**, **willow bark**, and **feverfew**.

- When making **rose hip** tea, take 10 whole hips (fresh or dry) and mash or break them open. Add 1 1/2 cups of very hot water (just before a boil is reached), and steep for 6–8 minutes.

    - Strain very well, as rose hips have irritating hairs within them.

- Other drinks and food you could consider include **pineapple juice** (for the bromelain), **apple cider vinegar** (can also be applied to muscle undiluted), **tart cherry juice** (twice a day for up to 3 weeks), and adding more **garlic** to your foods.

    - Consider adding foods that are rich in magnesium.

- **Devil's claw** can be purchased over the counter as a supplement or made into a tincture. Use no more than 15–20 drops from a tincture 2–3 times daily.

- Infused oils that can assist include **arnica** and **cannabis**. Other topical treatments include fresh **onion juice**, **capsaicin salve** (Chapter 7), and **devil's claw** salve.

- Don't forget about soaking in a relaxing **Epsom salt bath**.

Recipe

The only thing better than a massage is the ointment that adds a healing effect.

Muscle Soothing Ointment (*All Natural Pain Relief Salve*, n.d.)

Ingredients:

- 10 drops peppermint essential oil
- 10 drops lavender essential oil
- 1/4 c beeswax pastilles
- 1/4 c coconut oil

Directions:

1. Melt the beeswax over medium heat in a double boiler before adding the coconut oil.
2. Remove the mixture from the heat and let it cool for a few minutes before dripping in the essential oils.
3. Stir the mixture well before pouring it into a clean container.
4. Use as required when in pain.

Alternatives you could consider include acupuncture, mindful meditation, heat and cold treatments, yoga, or massage. If recovering from an old injury, you may want to make use of a physiotherapist or a chiropractor, depending on the injury type.

Gentle exercise is encouraged, as this can help strengthen muscles, bones, and joints while releasing endorphins. However, it's important to listen to your body and to stop when the pain starts.

Speak to your doctor if the pain is extreme enough to affect daily life, as there is a chance the injury may be worse than you suspect.

Sprains

Sprains occur when a limb is stretched, causing damage to ligaments, tendons, and other soft tissues. These sprains can vary from mild to severe. The general symptoms include limited movement, pain, bruising, redness, heat, swelling, and difficulty putting weight on the affected limb if knees and ankles are affected.

Remedies

Depending on the severity of the injury, a sprain can be treated at home, though a doctor's visit may be necessary to determine if there's severe damage that requires surgery or physiotherapy.

- Rest, ice, compression, and elevation (**RICE**) techniques will help elevate symptoms from the moment a sprain occurs. With less swelling, it's easier to see the extent of the injury.
- Help lower inflammation by eating **pineapple** as the bromelain reduces inflammation.

- Try a variety of inflammation and pain-reducing teas, such as **willow bark** and **turmeric**.

- Apply topical remedies such as **arnica-infused oil**, **cottonwood bud-infused oil** (also known as the balm of Gilead), **St. John's wort** (tea, compress, poultice, and infused oil), **witch hazel extract**, **lavender** (essential oil), **comfrey** (compress in Chapter 6, poultice, and infused oil), **yarrow** (compress, bath, and poultice), **California bay** (essential oil).

    - A **yarrow bath** is prepared with 1/3 ounce of dried yarrow added to your bath.

Recipes

The following recipes can help reduce the pain and inflammation associated with a sprain, but can also be used to treat other injuries.

Sprained Ankle Salve (*Easy Arnica Salve*, n.d.)
Ingredients:

- 1/2 oz beeswax

- 2 oz arnica-infused oil

- 1/2 tsp vitamin E oil (optional)

Directions:

1. Add the beeswax and infused oil to a double boiler and raise the temperature to medium. Stir as the wax melts.

2. Once melted, remove from the heat and add optional vitamin E.

3. Stir well and pour the salve into waiting containers.

4. The salve can be used as needed to treat bruises, sprains, strains, and any other niggling injuries.

Sprain Butter (*Comfrey Oil and Balm Recipes*, n.d.)
Ingredients:

- 5 drops tea tree essential oil
- 1/2 tsp vitamin E oil
- 1/2 c comfrey-infused oil
- 2 c shea butter
- 30-40 drops floral essential oil (lavender, rose, and so on)

Directions:

1. Heat the shea butter over low heat until liquid. Transfer to a heat-proof container.

2. Stir in the comfrey-infused oil and vitamin E.

3. After a few minutes, the mixture should start solidifying but still have a soft consistency.

4. Add in the essential oils.

5. Either hand whip or use an electrical beater to whip the mixture for 2–3 minutes.

6. Scoop the contents into the waiting containers to be used as needed.

See your doctor if the pain doesn't alleviate after using home treatments for a week, you can't move the joint or limb, the limb is best at an odd angle, the pain is severe, and the swelling doesn't go down after 2–3 days with treatment, or this is an injury that has occurred before.

If surgery is unnecessary, your doctor may suggest alternative therapies such as acupuncture, physiotherapy, or chiropractic.

Musculoskeletal injuries aren't the only miscellaneous injuries that can occur. In the following chapter, we'll discover remedies that treat common miscellaneous issues.

Chapter 15: Miscellaneous Remedies

Various ailments occur that we don't want to bother a doctor with, especially if they occur frequently with your family. Common miscellaneous problems include earaches, pink eye, and mouth sores (ulcers or cankers). For other ailments that may not appear here, refer to Chapter 6 for the first aid remedies.

Earaches

Earaches are often described as a burning, dull, or sharp pain in one or both ears. The pain is associated with a build-up of fluid that can't drain and becomes infected. For some people, it is a nuisance; for others, it is a debilitating pain. Earaches can occur for various reasons, some of which have nothing to do with the ear itself. Some common causes of earache are sinusitis, toothache, tooth grinding, post-nasal drip, sore throat, swimmer's ear, and many other causes. An earache's symptoms are pain, hearing loss, possibly some discharge, feeling ill, and fever.

Remedies

Before putting any remedy in your ear canal, speak to your doctor, as you don't want to cause excess pressure that could damage the eardrum inadvertently. Similarly, if a young child suffers an earache with a fever, take them to a doctor immediately. For adults, here are some remedies you can consider using.

- **Hot** and **cold compresses** can help with inflammation. Try 10 minutes with each treatment to the outside of the ear, or choose one temperature if that's more comfortable.
- Gargling **salt water** could help deal with infections in the eustachian tubes that connect the ears to the throat.
- Bake the **onion** at 450 °F for 15 minutes before cutting it in half and holding it close to your ear. Alternatively, juice the baked onion and apply the juice around the ear.
- Slightly warmed **olive oil** can be dripped into the ear canal. Ensure the oil is at or below body temperature. Tea tree essential oil can be added.
    - **Sesame oil** can be used similarly. Drip a few drops of **avartani** (Indian screw tree) infused in sesame oil into the ear.
    - Alternatively, add a few **ajwain seeds** with a few **garlic cloves** and boil them in **sesame oil** for a few minutes. Strain and drip a few drops of lukewarm oil in the ear.
- Apply some freshly squeezed **ginger juice** or **ginger-infused oil** to the *outside* of the ear canal. This can also be done with **crushed garlic** mixed into coconut oil or **garlic-infused oil**.
- Crush fresh **tulsi**, strain the juice, and drip 1–2 drops in the ear canal.
- Drip 1–2 drops of warmed **mullein-infused oil** into the ear canal.

- Adding some 10% **hydrogen peroxide** on a Q-tip to the outside of the ear canal can help kill off pathogenic microorganisms.

- Make a 1:1 ratio between **apple cider vinegar** and warm water before dipping a cotton ball in it. Squeeze excess fluid out and place it against the ear opening, leaving it there for a while. White vinegar can also be used.

    - In the case of swimmer's ear, make a 1:1 ratio of **vinegar** to **rubbing alcohol** and add to the outside of the ear.

Don't be afraid to use pain remedies within this book or OTC painkillers if the pain is too much. You can also try to distract yourself from the pain.

Alternative therapies that could help include sleeping elevated and off of the affected ear, chewing on gum with changing elevations (effective when flying), acupressure, neck exercises, or a facial massage.

See a doctor when the pain is acute, you have a fever, the ear is draining (could be pus), and the symptoms continue to get worse. Other symptoms to look out for are swelling behind the ear, severe pain that suddenly stops (a sign that the ear drum has ruptured), facial muscles twitching, severe headaches, and dizziness.

Pink Eye (Conjunctivitis)

Pink eye is when the sclera (white part of the eye) becomes pink or red, swells, and becomes itchy or feels like it's burning. There are three types of pink eye: viral (produces watery tears), bacterial (produces pus), and allergic. The latter two are highly contagious. You may require a doctor to identify the type you have.

Remedies

To deal with pink eye, think about hygiene. Wash your hands thoroughly, don't touch your eyes unless cleaning them, and use antibacterial wipes on all surfaces you handle. Other than that, here are some remedies aimed at the different types of pink eye.

- Use **warm compresses** for viral and bacterial pink eye, but a **cold compress** for allergic pink eye.
    - For compresses, there are various teas you can use, such as **chamomile**, **echinacea**, and **astragalus**. These remedies can also be drunk.
    - **Echinacea** and **astragalus** can also be consumed as tinctures to improve immunity.
- Don't throw out your **black** or **green tea bags** after using them. Place them in the fridge for 20 minutes and then add them to your closed eyes for 30 minutes.
- Herbal washes can be made from teas that include **fennel**, **chamomile**, **eyebright**, **plantain**, and **marigold**.
    - An eye wash made of **saline** can also be used. Mix 2 cups of water with a teaspoon of salt and boil the mixture for 15 minutes. Allow cooling to room

temperature before using on eyes. This helps with allergic and viral pink eye.

- Add 3 drops of **rose water** to your eyes daily for 1–3 days (viral and allergic pink eye).
- **Turmeric** can be drunk as tea or a compress can be made. Add 2 tablespoons of powder to a cup of boiled water and allow it to steep for 5–10 minutes. Strain and apply with cotton balls to your closed eyes.
- Create a steam bath with essential oils such as **lavender**, **peppermint**, **eucalyptus**, and **myrrh**.
- Apply **coconut oil** 1–2 inches away from the eyes to relieve itchiness. This can also be done with **aloe vera** gel.
- To soothe the allergic pink eye, mix a 1:1 ratio of **milk** and **honey** before applying it with a dropper to the eyes.

  It's vital to identify the correct pink eye, as this remedy can worsen the symptoms in other varieties.
- **Cat's claw** and **eyebright** can be used as a wash or compress.
  - Take 0.035 ounces of cat's claw and simmer it for 20 minutes in a cup of water.
  - Allow it to steep a further 10 minutes before straining well and using it as an eyewash.
  - Use 1–3 teaspoons of eyebright in a cup of water, then allow it to steep for 30 minutes. Strain well if used for a wash.

Recipes

Soothe the annoying symptoms of any pink eye with the following recipes.

Pink Eye Poultice (Oliver, 2015)
Ingredients:

- 2 tbsp dried calendula blossoms
- 2 tbsp fennel seeds, crushed
- 2 c sterilized water
- 2 chamomile tea bags
- 1 tbsp honey

Directions:

1. Pour water into a saucepan and bring to the point of boil, then turn off the heat.
2. Add the tea bags, blossoms, and seeds to the water and allow them to steep for 10 minutes.
3. Remove the tea bags and squeeze most of the moisture out.
4. Wrap the bags in cheesecloth and apply the honey on one side of both bags.
5. Lie back and apply both bags, honey-side down, to your closed eyelids for 10–15 minutes.
6. This remedy can be applied twice a day.

Pink Eye Wash (Hentschel, 2016)
Ingredients:

- 1 part dried chamomile
- 1 part dried eyebright
- 2 c boiled water

Directions:

1. Mix the dried chamomile to the eyebright. Take 4 teaspoons of the mixture and add it to the boiled water. Allow the mixture to steep for 10 minutes.
2. Strain twice with a finely woven cloth or a coffee filter.
3. Pour the lukewarm wash into a sterile eyebath container or use an eye pad to soak up the herbal wash.
4. Apply remedy up to 4 times a day, throwing away pads or sterilizing the eyebath between uses. The remedy may sting a little.
5. Make a fresh batch every 12 hours.

Enrich your diet with garlic, zinc, probiotics, and vitamins A, B-complex, C, and K. These additions help improve your immune system, strengthening your body to tackle infections before they happen.

You can also use OTC eye drops to keep your eyes lubricated and reduce itchiness.

Reach out to your doctor if the symptoms don't clear up within a week with treatment if you experience light sensitivity, struggle to see, have a high fever, or if the affected eye(s) is painful.

Mouth Sores (Ulcers and Cankers)

Mouth sores are open patches of skin on the lips and inside the mouth. They are often painful and can make eating and drinking difficult.

Various causes of this ailment exist, such as sensitivities or intolerances to certain foods (citrus, gluten, strawberries, or pineapples), a lack of certain vitamins, stress, viral or bacterial responses, accidentally biting yourself, and possible oral cancers.

Remedies

Mouth sores of all kinds are easily treated at home, and here are a few remedies you can try to reduce the sores and alleviate the pain.

- Try topical applications such as **honey**, b**aking soda poultice**, **coconut oil**, **toothpaste**, **coconut milk** (3–4 times a day), **turmeric paste**, **garlic** (keep in place for 1–2 minutes), **milk of magnesia** (3 times a day), **aloe vera** gel, or **tulsi** poultice.
- Use **chamomile** tea bags as a compress, or dab some tea on the sores 3–4 times a day.
- Gargling **salt water** will assist in dealing with internal mouth sores.
- Chew on **cloves** or dab some clove essential oil in a carrier oil on the injury.
- There are various mouth rinses you can use.

    - Add a tablespoon of **apple cider vinegar** to 1/2 cup of warm water. Rinse the mouth for 1–2 minutes, then rinse with plain water. Use this remedy in the morning and evening.
    - Mix a teaspoon of **baking soda** with 1/2 cup of water. Swirl the mixture in your mouth for 15–30 seconds. Repeat every few hours.
    - Teas, such as **echinacea**, **sage**, **tulsi**, and **licorice root**, can be swirled in the mouth for about 2 minutes before spitting out.
- **Licorice root** can be powdered and applied to the sore directly.
- Apply 1–2 drops of **propolis extract** 4–5 times a day. Propolis is made by bees, so avoid this remedy if you're allergic to bees.
- Pour 1/4 cup of 10% **hydrogen peroxide** into 1/2 a cup of water, then mix. Use a cotton ball to apply the remedy to the affected area. The remedy is very bitter.

Recipe

Honey assists in healing, so store this salve away to use when affected by mouth sores.

Honey Healing Salve (*How to Make a Simple Healing Salve Recipe*, n.d.)
Ingredients:

- 1 part beeswax

- 2–3 teaspoons of honey
- 10 drops of your favorite essential oil
- 4 parts carrier oil of choice (such as coconut oil)

Directions:

1. Melt the wax in a double boiler over medium heat before pouring it into the carrier oil.
2. Mix well and then remove from the heat. Allow the mixture a few minutes to cool.
3. Drip in the essential oil and stir in the honey.
4. Decant into waiting containers and allow to solidify.
5. Use as required.

Orange juice is high in vitamin C, so include it in your diet. You can also cook and puree cabbage, drinking 1/2 a cup 3–4 times daily. Don't forget to add probiotics to your diet to help fight infections from the inside and boost immunity.

See your doctor if there is no improvement in a mouth sore after 5–7 days with treatment, the sore is redder and swollen (possible bacterial infection), doesn't respond to any treatments, occurs at the same time as a fever, or more sores develop before the old ones are healed.

While there are many other miscellaneous ailments, this is a great opportunity to gather the necessary research and develop your own chapter in your medicinal remedy notebook!

Now, turn to the next chapter to look at ways herbal remedies can help with detoxing. There's a reason I dedicated an entire chapter to this topic—it's that *important*.

Chapter 16: Detox

Detoxing cleans the body of unwanted toxins, often caused by modern living and diet. Generally, a detox is done through a change in diet. A change in diet can be as extreme as a short-term juicing diet or a lifetime commitment to adopting an anti-inflammatory diet.

The body's filtration and detoxification organs include the kidneys, lymphatic system, skin, liver, and digestive tract. Diet changes can help support these organs in removing unwanted substances from the body. Before undertaking extreme detoxing practices, speaking to a doctor or nutritionist is best to prevent possible nutritional imbalances.

If you're suffering from unexplained fatigue, headaches, insomnia, weight gain, skin breakouts, and even mood swings, it may be a sign that you need to consider doing a detox.

Remedies

Many bitter herbs have been used for centuries to support detoxification and overall stomach health by supporting and nurturing detoxing organs. Here are a few remedies to improve the strength of your detoxing organs.

- Tea is a great way to work detoxing herbs into your diet. Consider using teas that contain **red clover**, **dandelion**, **stinging nettle**, **milk thistle** (Chapter 9), **turmeric**, **calendula**, **green tea**, **ginger**, and **tulsi**.

- A great liver support is **Schisandra berry**, especially if you take it in the morning. Take 1–2 tablespoons of the dried berries and allow them to simmer with 2 cups of water covered for 15–20 minutes.
    - Schisandra berry can replace hibiscus in other tea blends and pairs well with rosehips, hawthorn, and elderberry. Alternatively, chew on a few dried berries.
- **Burdock** tea and tincture help support the liver. Take 1.7–3.5 ounces of dried root and boil it with 4 cups of water for 10–15 minutes. Strain and sweeten with honey. Alternatively, take burdock tincture. Up to 3 times a day, take 10–20 drops in a glass of water. You can find the recipe below.
- Create a **blessed thistle**, also known as holy thistle, tea by steeping 1–3 teaspoons of dried stems, leaves, or flowers in a cup of boiled water for 5–15 minutes.
- Collect a cup of fresh **white pine** needles with the sheaths at the base removed, and add a quart of boiled water over them. Allow them to steep for 20 minutes and sweeten after straining. Note that not all pine species are edible.
- **Chlorella** and **spirulina** are algae that support detoxing organs and can be found in many supplement forms in pharmacies. The dosage will depend on the product.
- A **bentonite clay** bath soak is perfect to soak away your stresses and toxins. Place 1–3 cups in a bathtub with hot water and soak for 10–20 minutes. It's a good idea to start with a cup of clay as it can affect sensitive skin.

- Try an **elecampane** decoction by adding 2 tablespoons of dried root to 1–2 cups water and simmering for 20 minutes. Honey will be needed to sweeten it. Alternatively, take 0.06–0.1 ounces of elecampane tincture 2–3 times daily.

- **Yellow dock** can be used as a tea or a tincture. For the tea, take 1–2 teaspoons of dried root and boil it in 2 cups of water for 10 minutes. Use 1/4–1/2 teaspoon of the tincture 3 times daily.

- A **cleavers** infusion makes for a wonderful morning pick-me-up. Take a handful of fresh cleavers, wash them, and chop them roughly before adding them to a large jug with water. Cover the jug and keep it on the counter overnight. The following day, strain the liquid and add it to the fridge for a few hours before enjoying it like a summer drink.

You can also consider adding cilantro to your diet. However, note that not everyone enjoys the taste of fresh cilantro, as it may taste like soap to them.

Recipes

There are many ways to detox your system by bolstering the strength of your detoxing organs. Below is a mixture of tea blends, decoctions, oxymels, and more for you to try.

Bitter Root Tea (Groves, 2021)

Ingredients:

- 16 oz water

- 1 tsp dried dandelion root
- 1 tsp dried chicory root
- 1 tsp dried burdock root

Directions:

1. Add the dried herbs to a saucepan with the water, then simmer for 15 minutes.
2. Strain and store in the fridge until ready to use.

Nettle-Clover Infusion (Groves, 2021)

Ingredients:

- 1/2 oz dried nettles
- 1/2 oz dried red clover blossoms
- 1 qt boiled water
- 1/4 oz dried peppermint leaves (optional)
- 1/4 oz dried violet leaves (optional)

Directions:

1. Add the dried herbs to the boiled water and allow it to steep covered for at least 4 hours. If you wish, you can let the mixture steep overnight.
2. Strain and enjoy the tea.

Ginger-Dandelion Oxymel (Groves, 2021)

Ingredients:

- 1 part dried ginger roots, roughly chopped
- 1 part dried dandelion roots, roughly chopped
- apple cider vinegar
- honey

Directions:

1. Add the dried herbs to fill half the jar you're using.
2. Pour in the vinegar and honey to create a 3:1 ratio. Add more honey if you prefer a sweeter oxymel.
3. Close and shake to ensure everything is well coated.
4. Allow it to steep in a cool, dark location for 2 weeks, shaking daily.
5. Strain through cheesecloth and transfer the oxymel to a clean container.
6. Take 1/4–1/2 teaspoon with each meal or use it as a tangy salad dressing.

Detox Concentrated Tea (Bomgren, 2023)

Ingredients:

- 1–2 tsp ground cinnamon

- 5–6-in fresh ginger, peeled and sliced thinly
- 1 tsp ground turmeric
- 6 c water
- juice of 6 freshly squeezed lemons
- 1/2 tsp cayenne pepper (optional)

For serving

- juice of 1/2 lemon
- 6 oz water

Directions:

1. Add the ginger slices to the water and lemon juice in the saucepan.
2. Bring the mixture to a boil and then lower to a simmer for 10 minutes.
3. Add turmeric, cinnamon, and optional cayenne to the simmering mixture and continue to simmer for another 10 minutes.
4. Strain well and place in the fridge for later use, or enjoy warm.
5. This is a concentrated tea and should be watered down before use. Use 1/4 cup of the mixture and add it to 6 ounces of water (hot or cold) with the juice of half a lemon.

Floral and Green Detox Tea (Feiereisen, 2022)

Ingredients:

- 10 oz water
- 3 thin slices fresh ginger root, peeled
- 1 tbsp rose buds
- 1 tbsp stinging nettle
- 1 tbsp dandelion root

Directions:

1. Allow all the ingredients to steep in the freshly boiled water for 15 minutes.
2. Steep well before sipping.

Detox Drink (Feiereisen, 2022)

Ingredients:

- 3–4 lime slices
- 3–4 lemon slices
- 8 oz water
- 3–4 sprigs fresh mint
- some cucumber slices

Directions:

1. Add the ingredients to a jug with the water and allow them to steep for several hours before serving.

Liver Detox Tincture (Dessinger, 2022)

Ingredients:

- 12 1/2 ounces 100 proof alcohol
- 1/4 oz dried turmeric root
- 1/2 oz dried burdock root
- 1 oz dried milk thistle seed
- 1/2 oz dried dandelion root
- 1/4 oz dried organic artichoke leaf (optional)

Directions:

- Use your pestle and mortar to grind the milk thistle seeds coarsely.
- Add all the roots and seeds to a quart-sized jar, then pour over the alcohol.
- Shake the contents to ensure everything is soaked through before storing the jar in a cool, dark place for the next 3–5 weeks. Shake now and again.
- Strain the tincture through some cheesecloth, retaining the liquid.

- Decant the tincture into amber-colored dropper bottles.
- Use 1/2–1 teaspoon of the tincture 2–3 times daily before any meals are taken.

Burdock Tincture (Rose, 2023)

Ingredients:

- 6 oz dried burdock root, coarsely chopped
- 12 oz Vodka

Directions:

1. Add the burdock root to a glass container and add the alcohol.
2. Give a shake and ensure the root pieces are below the alcohol level before storing the jar in a cool, dark place.
3. Allow the tincture to steep for 4–6 weeks, shaking the contents daily. Top up alcohol as needed.
4. Once ready, strain the tincture through cheesecloth before adding the liquid to amber-colored bottles.

While detoxing is safe for most people, if you have diabetes or any other medical condition, it's a good idea to work with your doctor to determine how to go about your detoxing period.

The whole point of detoxing is to support your body and the various detoxing organs in doing their job. You can assist by improving your diet, cutting out addictive substances (such as smoking and drinking), getting enough sleep, engaging in moderate exercise, and relaxing to help reduce stress. If your body works optimally, it removes any toxins that shouldn't be in it.

In the following chapter, we'll examine how you can improve your overall well-being through various herbal remedies.

Chapter 17: General Well-Being

A person's general well-being is feeling good about themselves and functioning normally in all day-to-day activities. This isn't only about the physical body, but also your mental and emotional control, giving you a sense of purpose. While everyone suffers a down day from time to time, there are many ways you can improve your energy, cognitive function, immunity, and mood.

Boosting Energy and Fighting Fatigue

Everyone has woken up with the Monday blues, where they don't want to get up and go to work. Yet, it's more than not having the will to get up and do anything; there doesn't seem to be any energy to do anything you used to do with gusto.

The causes of fatigue are numerous, but the general culprits are poor sleep, unmanaged stress, unbalanced or poor diet, too much caffeine, alcohol, lack of exercise, and so much more.

Remedies

Before you reach for something with caffeine, realize that you could be setting yourself up for failure. Excess caffeine use can cause increased blood pressure, heart rate, anxiety, and nervousness. Thankfully, there are many ways to improve your energy without exceeding your moderate daily intake of caffeine.

- Rather than starting your day with coffee, try tea instead. Consider teas that include **ashwagandha**, **Rhodiola** (Chapter 8), **green tea**, **ginseng**, **tulsi**, **Schisandra**, **peppermint**, **ginger**, **lemon balm**, **rosemary**, **sage**, **ginkgo** (Chapter 8), and **astragalus**.

- Sniffing **peppermint** essential oil will give you the boost you need to get through your day.

- **Forskolin**, coleus root, can be enjoyed as a tea with 1/2–1 teaspoon dried leaves steeped in a cup of hot water for 5 minutes before steeping.

- **French oak** tea may be bitter, but it may be the wake-up call you need. Take a teaspoon of the dried bark and stereo it in a cup of boiled water for at least 10 minutes. The longer you steep, the more bitter the drink will become.

- **Sleuthero**, otherwise known as **Siberian ginseng**, tea is made with 1/2 tablespoon of dried root (or 1/2 teaspoon of ground root) that is simmered with a cup of water for 15 minutes. Remove from heat and steep for 30 minutes, or overnight, before straining and enjoying cool.

- While **gota kola** tea can help fight fatigue, don't drink more than 3 cups daily, and no longer than 6 weeks before taking a 2-week break. Add a teaspoon of the dried leaves to a cup of water, allowing it to steep for 10–15 minutes. This tea can be combined with tulsi or ginkgo.

Recipes

Try some of the following recipes to give you the required boost of energy and strength to fight fatigue.

Energy Boosting Decoction (Gibson, 2023)
Ingredients:

- 2 tbsp dried ashwagandha root
- 3 tbsp dried hibiscus
- 3 tbsp dried green tea leaves
- 1 tbsp dried peppermint
- 2 tbsp dried orange peel

Directions:

1. Blend the dried herbs and place them in an airtight container.
2. When ready to enjoy the blend, add 2 tablespoons of the mixture to 1 1/2 cups of water in a saucepan.
3. Bring the water to a boil, then reduce the temperature to a simmer. Cover the saucepan and continue to simmer for 15–20 minutes.
4. Once the simmer is complete, strain the tea through cheesecloth.
5. Enjoy the tea while it is still hot.

Energized Almonds (Herbal Academy, 2015)
Ingredients:

- 1 tsp fresh thyme, finely chopped
- 2 c almonds (ALLERGY ALERT)
- 1 tbsp olive oil

- 1/2 c maple syrup or honey
- 1 tsp fresh rosemary, finely chopped
- 1 tsp fresh oregano, finely chopped
- pinch of salt

Directions:

1. Preheat oven to 350 °F.
2. Add all the ingredients on a rimmed baking sheet and mix until the nuts are well coated.
3. Bake in the oven, occasionally shifting the nuts until they are golden brown. This can take from 8–20 minutes.
4. The recipe makes 2 cups of nuts, and a portion is a 1/4 cup. Store the nuts in an airtight container in a cool, dark place.

Ginger and Cardamon Tea (5 *Ways to Make Natural Energy Drink*, 2020)
Ingredients:

- 2 thin slices of fresh ginger
- 1/4 tsp turmeric powder
- 1 cup hot water
- juice from a 1/2-inch fresh ginger piece
- 1/4 tsp ground cardamom
- 1–2 tsp honey

Directions:

1. Add all the ingredients and stir until the honey is dissolved.

2. Allow the mixture to steep for 5 minutes.

3. Strain and enjoy while still warm.

One of the main alternatives to fighting fatigue is improving your life in terms of exercise, diet, and hydration.

Sadly, fatigue can be the beginning signs of many illnesses. So, if you find that the fatigue doesn't improve after 2 weeks with changes to diet, hydration, exercise, and herbal remedies, it's time to chat with your doctor.

Tell them what you have been trying so they can make educated suggestions moving forward.

Boosting Focus, Memory, and Cognitive Function

Whether trying to concentrate on your job or preparing for a test, the last thing you want is for your brain to turn on you suddenly. A lack of focus can be caused by stress, anxiety, depression, insomnia, health problems, some medications, hormonal changes, and exhaustion (mental and physical).

If your brain can't focus, it causes problems with cognition and memory.

Remedies

Losing focus can result in mistakes in your work, accidents, brain fog, difficulty making decisions, difficulty remembering (even from a few hours ago), and more. Rein your brain to do what you expect of it through the use of the following remedies.

- Boost your brain's function with teas that contain **sage**, **turmeric** (try the turmeric latte in the recipe section), **ginkgo**, **ashwagandha**, **ginseng**, **gotu kola**, **lemon balm**, **rosemary**, **peppermint**, **eleuthero root**, **tulsi**, **chamomile**, **green tea**, **Rhodiola**, **cinnamon**, **nutmeg**, and **thyme**.
- The sense of smell in the brain is closely linked to memory, so make use of essential oils such as **rosemary** and **peppermint** when learning.
- **Brahmi** (*Bacopa monnieri*) can be used to make a brain tonic by adding 1/2 a teaspoon of the dried herb together with 1/2 teaspoon of dried ashwagandha saucepan with 1/2 cup of water and 1/2 cup milk. Bring the mixture to a low simmer and keep it there for 15 minutes. Strain and enjoy in the morning and evening.
- **Wood betony** tea can be made with 1–2 teaspoons of dried flowers or leaves that are steeped in a cup of boiled water for 15 minutes. Enjoy 1–2 cups daily.
- You can also enjoy 5–10 drops of **cayenne** tincture up to 2 times daily or dust the spice over your food.

Recipes

Consider some of the following recipes to bring your brain into focus, allowing it to concentrate and retain information more readily.

Brain Tonic Tea (Herbal Academy, 2019b)
Ingredients:

- 2 c water, boiled
- 2 tbsp dried spearmint
- 2 tsp dried sage
- 1 tbsp dried tulsi

Directions:

1. Add the dried herbs to a container and then pour over the boiled water.
2. Cover the container and allow the mixture to steep for 5–20 minutes, depending on how strong you like the tea.
3. Strain the herbs and squeeze any excess liquid from them.
4. Enjoy 1–2 cups of tea about 30 minutes before you start studying to get the best from your activated brain cells.

Turmeric Latte (Shoemaker, 2020)
Ingredients:

- 1 1/2 tsp ground turmeric
- 2 cups milk or plant-based milk
- cinnamon powder (optional)
- honey or stevia (optional)
- ground black pepper (optional)

Directions:

1. Heat the milk over low temperature until it's hot.
2. Add the turmeric and whisk it into the milk before removing the mixture from the heat.
3. Pour the mixture into 2 mugs and add optional ingredients before enjoying.

Your ability to focus also relies on what you put into your body. Add a variety of fruits and vegetables (particularly green types), saffron, kombucha, and fruit juices such as blueberry and orange.

If you find that losing focus and memory loss are starting to affect your life, it's time to talk to your doctor.

Improving Mood

Everyone feels down from time to time, especially during colder months. While it may be a feeling of melancholy to some, to others, it can be as bad as seasonal affective disorder (S.A.D.). There is no reason to leave yourself feeling down in the dumps.

Remedies

Pick yourself up with a range of remedies that are sure to improve your mood and make your day a little brighter.

- A change in diet is a great way to improve your mood. Include foods, such as **garlic**, **honey**, **saffron**, **nutmeg**, and **cinnamon**.
- If you're taking strain at work or under emotional stress, try some teas containing **St John's wort**, **lemon balm**, **hawthorn** (Chapter 7), **ashwagandha**, **turmeric**, **fennel**, **lemongrass**, **peppermint**, **cinnamon**, **ginger**, **clove** (Chapter 9), **thyme**, **nutmeg**, **Rhodiola**, **tulsi**, **licorice**, and **ginseng**.
- You can also boost your mood by smelling essential oils such as **lavender**, **peppermint**, **rosemary**, **orange**, **bergamot**, **ylang-ylang**, **lemon**, **mimosa**, and **neroli**.
- Add some frozen **raspberries** to a cup of hot water and allow them to thaw before crushing them and enjoying the drink.
- **Velvet bean** (*Mucuna pruriens*) is said to perk people up. This remedy is sold as a supplement but can also be found in some chai drinks. Powdered mucuna is readily sold as a drink enhancer.

If nothing manages to lift your mood and you have been feeling down for a while, it may be time to speak to a professional who can help determine the problem.

Improving the Immune System

It's likely you already know the signs of a poor immune system. It's more than frequent infections or illnesses. If your immune system isn't functioning correctly, common symptoms can range from fever, stomach or digestive issues, rashes, fatigue, unexplained wounds, headaches, and always feeling ill.

Remedies

If your immune system is in peak condition, it does all the heavy lifting, keeping your body functioning as it should. Many herbs and herbal remedies boost your immune system and give your body a fighting chance before you notice signs of illness.

- Include ingredients such as **paprika**, **maitake** (hen-of-the-wood), **reishi** mushrooms, and **garlic** in your meals for their various health benefits.
- Teas such as **turmeric**, **echinacea**, **ginger**, **cinnamon**, **peppermint**, **astragalus**, **elderberry**, **goldenseal** (Chapter 11), **olive leaf** (Chapter 7), **oregano**, **ashwagandha**, **ginseng**, **tulsi**, and **licorice** boost various parts of the body's immune system.

    - Elderberry tea for immune support should be made with 2–4 tablespoons of dried berries in a cup of hot water, steeping for 15 minutes before drinking.
    - A cinnamon paste can be made with a teaspoon of honey and 1/2 a teaspoon of cinnamon before dissolving in a cup of hot water to drink.

- If you're not allergic to bees, try **propolis** supplements or tinctures. 10 drops of propolis tincture in a shot glass of water can be gargled and then swallowed.
- **Andrographis** tea can be made with a teaspoon of dried herb in a cup of hot water. Allow it to steep for 10–15 minutes and then drink on an empty stomach.
- **Grindelia**, also known as gumweed, tea is made with 2 tablespoons of dried herb, steeped in a quart of hot water covered for 10 minutes. Enjoy 2–3 cups daily.
- Even smelling essential oils such as **peppermint** and **eucalyptus** can boost your immune system.

Recipes

A strong immune system keeps your body in a condition to keep you healthy and functioning at your best. Here are a few recipes to help you.

Immune Boosting Bitters (La Forge, 2020)

Ingredients:

- 10 oz 100% proof alcohol

- 1 tsp dried ginger
- 2 tsp boiled water
- 1 tbsp honey
- 1 tsp cardamom seeds
- 1 cinnamon stick
- 1 oz dried astragalus root
- 1 oz dried angelica root
- 1 tsp dried orange peel
- 1/2 oz dried chamomile

Directions:

1. Add the honey to the boiling water to dissolve it. All the mixture to cool.
2. Place the dissolved honey, with the herbs and spices, in a mason jar before topping up with alcohol.
3. Seal the jar and place it in a cool, dark location for 2–4 weeks. Shake daily, topping up alcohol as needed.
4. After steeping, strain the tincture through cheesecloth.
5. Transfer the tincture to a dark-colored container. Store away from direct sunlight and heat.
6. Add a few drops to your tea when flu season starts to help boost your immune system.

Fire Cider

Ingredients:

- apple cider vinegar
- 1 part garlic, crushed or finely chopped
- 1/2 part fresh ginger, grated
- 1 part onion, chopped finely
- 1 part horseradish, chopped finely
- pinch of cayenne (more if you like spicy)
- honey to taste

Directions:

1. After preparing the horseradish, onion, and garlic, allow them to sit for 5–10 minutes. This helps to activate their constituents.
2. Add these to a jar together with the ginger, ensuring they fill half the volume.
3. Squeeze in enough honey to form a thick layer over the mixture, and then add the apple cider vinegar to be 2–3 inches above that.
4. Sprinkle in the cayenne before sealing the container and giving the mixture a shake.
5. Store the mixture for 2–4 weeks, shaking now and again.
6. Strain the solids from the fire cider and pour the retained liquid into a clean container.

7. Store in the fridge and take a shot of the mixture if the unpleasant tickle starts in your throat.

Anti-Infection Tincture Mixture

Ingredients:

- 1/2 part licorice root tincture
- 1 part Oregon grape root tincture
- 1/2 part usnea tincture
- 1 part ginger root tincture
- 2 parts echinacea root tincture
- 2 parts echinacea leaf and flower tincture

Directions:

1. This recipe requires the tinctures to be made separately and then combined after the infusion process is complete.

Herbal Tea Immune Boost

Ingredients:

- 1 tbsp dried lemon balm
- 1 qt water
- 1/8 tsp dried lemon peel
- 2 tbsp dried astragalus
- 1 tbsp dried ginger
- honey to taste

Directions:

1. Add the water, astragalus, lemon peel, and ginger to a saucepan and simmer covered for 20 minutes.

2. Remove from heat, add in the lemon balm, cover, and steep for another 20 minutes.

3. The tea should be enjoyed hot with a splash of honey. The mixture will last up to 24 hours in the fridge.

Hygiene is your best bet for improving your immunity. By washing your hands and avoiding others who are sick, you'll prevent yourself from picking up illness, which could impact your immunity, making it easier for other infections to overtax your immune system.

If infections or the previously mentioned symptoms persist, become more frequent, or worsen despite home treatments, there may be an underlying cause. Speak to your doctor or another health professional to determine your next steps.

While general well-being is important, how you look and feel about it can significantly impact you mentally and emotionally. Let's move on to the bonus chapter.

Chapter 18: Remedies For Beauty

Beauty may be in the eye of the beholder, but that isn't only for strangers who look at you. If you're at peace with how you look, this helps to boost your confidence and self-esteem, both of which affect your mental and emotional health.

Softer, Glowing Skin

Everyone loves the feel and look of healthy skin. Your skin is worth pampering, not just looking after when something goes wrong.

Remedies

While there are many remedies to beautify skin, a few use similar ingredients that have already been discussed.

- Try some topical treatments such as **avocado** (mash the fruit and apply it, washing it away after 15 minutes), **aloe vera** gel, **olive oil**, **shea butter**, **turmeric paste**, **coconut oil**, and even **yogurt** (wash off after 10–15 minutes).
- An **oatmeal** bath will do wonders for your skin, but so will a milk bath. Add 2–3 cups of milk to your bath and soak for 10–15 minutes. You can also add essential oils like lemon and rose to the bath water.

- Make a facial scrub of equal parts **sugar** and **coconut oil**. Scrub gently and wash your face well.
- Try a **lemon** and **honey** mask. Mix 1 part honey to 1 part lemon juice, mix, then apply to your skin for 15–20 minutes before rinsing.
- When softening facial skin, you can consider **orange** juice, orange peel paste, or a green tea compress.
    - To make an orange peel paste, take a few pieces of orange peel and a few drops of rose water and blend until a paste is formed. Apply to the face before rinsing away after 15 minutes.

The condition of your skin is influenced by the environment (especially the sun), hydration, sleep, and toxins such as smoke. Getting enough sleep and adequate hydration will improve your skin condition. Don't forget to cover up or use appropriate sunblock when out and about.

Reduce Eye Puffiness

Many factors and situations can cause eye puffiness. Allergies, exhaustion, crying, genetics, age, water retention, and even stress can affect the severity of puffiness.

Remedies

While nothing can be done about genetics or getting older, many remedies can be used to reduce the appearance of puffiness under the eyes.

- If you have a spare 10–15 minutes, there are many topical applications you can use. The most common is **cold compresses**, but you can also use **cucumber** or **potato** slices (up to 20 minutes), **aloe vera**, or cooled **black tea** bags.

- Add cotton balls with **rosewater** to closed eyes for 10–15 minutes.

- **Turmeric** paste can be applied under the eyes and left on for 10–15 minutes before needing to be rinsed. This remedy will stain.

- **Witch hazel** extract can be used the same way as rosewater but for only 5–10 minutes. This can be applied several times throughout the day, but be careful not to get any in your eyes.

- A gentle massage with some preferred carrier oil will also do wonders.

Eye puffiness can also be a sign of too much screen time, so cut back on that, especially at night. You can even add some parsley to your diet.

Teeth Whitening

Many people are embarrassed at their stained teeth and spend a fortune on whitening toothpaste or chemical treatments when it isn't required. Don't let stained teeth affect the way you feel about yourself.

Remedies

It's likely that you already have many of the ingredients found within these remedies to help whiten teeth. There are many to choose from, so pick those that best suit your tastes. It's vital that none of these remedies be swallowed and that you rinse your mouth well.

- **Baking soda** can be combined with crushed strawberries or lemon juice to make a paste. Brush for 2 minutes before spitting and rinsing.
- Melt some **coconut oil** and swirl it in your mouth for 5–20 minutes. This can also be done with olive oil or sesame oil.
- Dip the bristles of a wet toothbrush in some **activated charcoal**. Brush for 2 minutes, and then rinse your mouth thoroughly.
- Take 1/4 teaspoon of **apple cider vinegar**, and mix it in a cup of water. Gargle the mixture before brushing your teeth normally. Use this remedy 2–3 times weekly. This can also be done with neem tea as a gargle.
- Rub the white part of a **banana peel** against your teeth for 1–2 minutes.
- Add 2–3 drops of **orange essential oil** to the toothpaste on your brush before brushing. Use this remedy daily for a week.
- Dust your toothpaste with 1/8 teaspoon of ground **turmeric** before brushing for 2–3 minutes.

- Add **Epsom salts** to water in a 1:1 ratio, stir to dissolve, and then brush with this liquid. Afterward, gargle with the remaining liquid before rinsing the mouth with fresh water.

- Mix a teaspoon of **salt** with 2 teaspoons of **lemon juice** to make a paste. Brush your teeth with this paste twice a week.

- **Guava leaves** can be crushed into a paste and rubbed into teeth for 1–2 minutes before rinsing your mouth and brushing normally. Do this remedy on alternating days.

Teeth are stained by what we eat and drink. Reduce consumption of foods that stain while eating more fresh fruits and vegetables. These foods are abrasive and will help scrub your teeth clean. Enjoy some pineapple, as this will also help whiten your teeth.

Hair Care

Hair, like skin, can be affected by the environment or the toxins you're exposed to. Even the use of incorrect shampoos too often can affect the health of your hair.

Remedies

If you notice your hair is thinning, becoming brittle, or simply lacking the luster it once had, try some of the following remedies to improve it.

- Hair oils have been used for centuries to improve hair health. Create infused oils with oils such as **wheat germ**,

jojoba, **coconut**, **sweet almond**, or **walnut**, with herbs such as **hibiscus**, **ginseng**, **brahmi**, **jatamansi** (made with the rhizome), and **tridax daisy**.

  - Alternatively, use essential oils, such as **peppermint** and **rosemary**, in a carrier oil.
  - **Castor oil** can also be applied to wet hair.

- You can even consider making hair salves using **tulsi**, **gooseberry**, **aloe vera**, or **gotu kola**.
- When rinsing rice, don't discard the water. Rinsing your hair with **rice water** is said to help with thickness and growth.
- Teas that contain **sage**, **chamomile**, **lemon balm**, **peppermint**, or **rosemary** can also be used as a hair rinse.

When applying salves and infused oils, it should be done to wet hair and can remain on the hair for at least 30 minutes or overnight. If you leave the oil overnight, wrap your head in a towel and wash the oil out in the morning. Apply these remedies twice a week.

Tea rinses should be applied after you wash your hair and can be done 1–2 times weekly.

Many different herbal remedies can be used for various ailments, yet they only work well if your body is in the correct state to receive the healing. In the following chapter, we'll discuss ways to help improve your life and give your body the chance to heal itself.

Chapter 19: Living a Good Life

While herbal remedies can improve your life, if your body isn't in the right state to receive that help, no remedy or even pharmaceutical drugs will effectively treat any ailments. To ensure that your body can reach a state where it can self-heal, it's important to look at your diet, hydration, physical activity, and sleep hygiene, among others.

Diet

A healthy diet can mean different things to different people, and if you find that you need a specific one for you, it's best to see a nutritionist. Ideally, a healthy diet is one where you get all the nutrients you need to function, grow, and remain healthy.

Food contains macronutrients (carbohydrates, protein, and fiber) and micronutrients (minerals and vitamins). Deciding what to eat can be tricky, but your body will respond better if you consume more whole and unprocessed foods.

When choosing carbohydrates, consider fruit, vegetables, and whole grains. If gluten-intolerant or sensitive, look at ancient grains, such as sorghum, millet, and quinoa, as examples of whole grains. Eat a variety of colorful fruits and vegetables, with more vegetable portions. While starchy vegetables (potatoes and corn) are delicious, have them infrequently in favor of other vegetables.

You're spoiled for choice when it comes to protein. Red meat can be enjoyed occasionally but should be eaten infrequently.

However, you can still enjoy fish, poultry, white meat, seafood, shellfish, and plant-based proteins.

Don't forget nuts, legumes, and seeds, as they can be added to cereals and salads to give them an extra crunch and boost of healthy fats. Carbohydrates and plant-based proteins give you the necessary fiber to support healthy bowel movements and the gut microbiome.

Fat is required by the body, but not all fats are good for you. Avoid fried food, but make an effort to use plant-based oils in cooking or drizzle over salads.

Include seeds, nuts, avocados, and oily fish in your diet to get the good fats in your diet. Aim to consume more poly and monounsaturated fats over saturated fats.

Moderation is key. Trying to avoid all foods labeled as "unhealthy" can be detrimental to your emotional and mental health. If you want that piece of cake, enjoy a smaller portion, and less frequently. Eventually, you'll wonder why you ever needed it.

Hydration

The majority of the human body is made of water, and most of its functions (temperature regulation, flushing toxins, maintaining blood pressure, and more) require it for it to run correctly.

Dehydration can happen in a matter of hours, resulting in headaches, dry mouth, and dark urine. Ignoring these signs will result in the body starting to shut down and organs being permanently damaged.

Age, gender, activity, weight, climate, and overall health determine how much water a person needs to drink per day to fight dehydration. Generally, it's accepted that people need to consume 91–125 ounces of liquid per day. As food and drink plays a role in this, 9–12 1/2 cups of liquid should likely be drunk.

Note that this is any liquid, including non-alcoholic beverages, tea, and coffee, and not just water. Don't forget to include some electrolytes if you're very active, as while sweating, you're also losing mineral salts. However, keep in mind that drinking too many caffeinated drinks and drinks with electrolytes will cause more harm than good.

Physical Activity

Physical activity isn't just about exercise; it's about getting your body moving, increasing your heart rate, and working up a slight sweat. Remember, excessive or vigorous exercise can increase inflammation, causing more problems than it solves.

However, activity is still needed, as it's a way to reduce risks of various health issues (cancer, high blood pressure, and even type 2 diabetes), maintain weight, increase longevity, manage chronic conditions, strengthen bones and muscles, and reduce inflammation (if at moderate intensity).

You don't need to spend hours in the gym if you're active for at least 30 minutes for the majority of your week, doing activities such as walking, swimming, hiking, tai-chi, and gardening. You can even include some strength exercises, such as body weight exercises (squats, lunges, and pushups), as well as balance (yoga or Pilates) and flexibility (stretching).

Sleep Hygiene

Sleep takes up to a third of our life, so why continue to do activities that jeopardize it? With the invention of electric lights, people have been staying up later and later, reducing the number of hours they sleep and affecting their ability to sleep well.

There are several ways you can improve your sleep hygiene to improve your chances of getting a better night's rest. Some changes you could consider are the following:

- Stick to a consistent sleeping schedule.
- Reduce caffeine intake 3–7 hours before going to sleep.
- Have a routine in place, such as showering, breathing exercises, or meditation before bed, to help you wind down and destress.
- Avoid any screen time up to an hour before bedtime.
- Have a comfortable sleeping environment. Keep your room to 60–67 °F, as noiseless as possible, and reduce any lights (including phone screens).
- Don't fight sleep. If you feel tired, go to sleep.
- If you don't fall asleep within 20 minutes, get up and do some light activity. Try reading in a low light until you feel tired.
- Avoid excess napping during the day. Keep it to no more than 30 minutes.

- Don't consume any large meals or do heavy exercise before bed.

- Ideally, only use your bedroom for sex and sleeping.

You can even include relaxing scents in your room to help induce sleep. Add some dried lavender, marjoram, lemon balm, or peppermint to a muslin bag and place it inside your pillow. The scents will encourage relaxation, allowing you to fall asleep more easily.

Like everything you have learned in this book, there is no reason to make all these changes at once, as this could be too stressful and unsustainable, making it more difficult to fall asleep. Consider making a few small changes daily to get into the rhythm of better sleep hygiene, and soon, you'll be enjoying a night of more restful and quality sleep.

Conclusion

Your body is made up of various parts that work together in harmony to maintain a delicate balance that allows it to self-heal. Disruptions in this balance can lead to potential illnesses and mental conditions and increase the risk of developing chronic conditions, such as persistent inflammation, type 2 diabetes, and certain cancers.

In the past, people around the world used herbal remedies to treat various ailments. As time progressed, the active ingredients in many of these herbal remedies were identified, manufactured, and made into pharmaceutical drugs, which are now available either by prescription or over the counter. While many herbal remedies are still readily available, they are rarely prescribed by those who aren't trained in the field.

Not everyone is comfortable with using pharmaceutical drugs for a variety of reasons, and so they turn to using the remedies of the past. The FDA hasn't stringently tested herbal remedies, so it's important to understand and use them safely. Ideally, discussing their use with a doctor, naturopath, or traditional healer is best to ensure nothing you're taking can interact.

Herbal remedies come in a variety of preparations, some lasting a few days to several years. Each remedy serves a unique function, and as you learn more about them and their ingredients, you will become more comfortable treating common ailments yourself.

Storing them correctly will allow you to have them on hand whenever you may need them, particularly in emergencies requiring first aid. When storing remedies for future use, ensure they are correctly labeled to ensure their correct usage, especially for those that have to infuse for several weeks.

Herbal remedies are useful in treating anything, from infection to bladder concerns to strains, and even enhance natural beauty. With over 1,000 remedies to treat different ailments, this only scratches the surface when it comes to treating ailments within the comfort of your own home.

Creating remedies from various botanicals is a lifelong journey, and you should strive to continually learn about the plants that offer their healing natures to you. Don't stop at just reading this book; a wide world of herbal remedies is still to be explored and learned from. Keep a notebook on hand to jot down anything exciting you may discover in the future.

Whether growing, foraging, or purchasing, ensure you use only the highest-quality and properly sourced ingredients in your remedies. Use the correct tools for the job, and observe recipes as you create and store them correctly.

Preventing ailments starts with taking charge of your body and giving it the nutrients it needs, as well as enough rest, hydration, physical activity, and destressing strategies. A healthy diet, full of anti-inflammatory foods and healthy fats with adequate hydration, is the best start to achieving harmony in your body. Follow this with moderate exercise concentrating on strength, balance, flexibility, and cardio, plus quality sleep, and you have the recipe for success.

There is no better time than right now to take your health into your own hands. While there are cases where you should be speaking to a medical professional, there are many ailments you can treat yourself. Continue to monitor your health and learn more about what Mother Nature has to offer with her healing plants. Take the knowledge you've gained in this book and start improving your life today. You have nothing to lose and only your health to improve. Your healthier future awaits!

Dear Reader

I reserved this special space to express my heartfelt gratitude. Not just for your time and support in reading this book—though I sincerely appreciate it—but for being the inspiration behind its creation. The ultimate purpose of any book is to be read, and as I write these pages, I feel honored to know that your hands will hold them one day.

I hope this book touches you in the ways I intended and brings about the change you seek. If it does, it would mean a lot to hear your thoughts—leaving an honest review or rating on Amazon would mean the world to me.

Once again, thank you,
Aveline Clarke

Claim Your Gifts

Simply scan the QR code below to access the audiobook version and video bonuses.

Want more?

Check out our top sellers:

Our journey together doesn't have to end here.

References

About Barbara. (n.d.). Barbara O'Neill. barbara-oneill.mykajabi.com/about

Academy of Culinary Nutrition. (2024, January 30). Fire cider recipe and more immune-supportive tincture tips. Meghan Telpner. meghantelpner.com/fire-cider-recipe-and-more-immune-supportive-tincture-tips/

Adamant, A. (2023, February 24). *Nasturtium tincture*. Practical Self Reliance. practicalselfreliance.com/nasturtium-tincture/

admin. (2017, October 1). *12 herbal remedies for depression and anxiety*. Mental Health Food. mentalhealthfood.net/13-herbs-for-treating-depression-and-anxiety/

Ajmera, R. (2024, January 29). 10 home remedies to get rid of dandruff naturally. Healthline. healthline.com/nutrition/ways-to-treat-dandruff

Alieta. (2017, March 2). Artichoke leaf bitters. *Mountain Rose Herbs*. blog.mountainroseherbs.com/artichoke-leaf-bitters

Alissa. (2016, December 16). Creating a herbal notebook. The Herbal Homeschool. theherbalhomeschool.com/2016/12/16/creating-a-herbal-notebook/

All natural pain relief salve recipe: How to make, best recipe. (n.d.). *Khela Herbs*. khelaherbs.com/blog/pain-relief-salve-recipe

Ames, H. (2023, December 14). Six effective herbs and remedies for asthma relief. Medical News Today. medicalnewstoday.com/articles/herbs-for-asthma-relief

Andrea. (n.d.). *Creating a kitchen pharmacy: Equipment and supplies*. Frugally Sustainable. frugallysustainable.com/creating-a-kitchen-pharmacy-equipment-and-supplies/

Andrographis. (n.d.). Good Food Store. goodfoodstore.com/Aisle7/Default.aspx?resource=%2Fassets%2Fnutritional-supplement%2Fandrographis%2Fhow-it-works

Are there alternative treatments for overactive bladder? (n.d.). WebMD. webmd.com/urinary-incontinence-oab/ss/slideshow-oab-natural-remedies

Asamoah, K. (2018, June 11). *7 home remedies for ear infections*. Express MD. expressmdcare.com/7-home-remedies-for-ear-infection/

Axe, J. (2022, January 28). *15 carrier oils for essential oils*. Dr. Axe. draxe.com/essential-oils/carrier-oils-for-essential-oils/

Axe, J. (2023, January 20). *DIY arthritis ointment for joint pain*. Dr. Axe. draxe.com/beauty/diy-arthritis-ointment/

Baillie, L. (n.d.). 5 top herbs for muscle and joint pain. A.Vogel. avogel.co.uk/health/muscles-joints/5-top-herbs-for-muscle-and-joint-pain/

Balick, M. J. (2016, December 13). 30 herbs that fight cold and flu. Prevention. prevention.com/health/g20493406/30-herbs-that-fight-cold-and-flu/

Balms, salves & ointments. (n.d.). Fragrant Earth Organics. fragrantearth.com/index.php?route=product/category&path=50_156

Barden, A. (2020, August 26). Can you "cure" pink eye naturally? All about Vision. allaboutvision.com/treatments-and-surgery/natural-remedies-pink-eye/

Barode, S. (2024a, January 10). Home remedies for vomiting. *PharmEasy*. pharmeasy.in/blog/home-remedies-for-vomiting/

Barode, S. (2024b, March 19). Simple home remedies for bloating. *PharmEasy*. pharmeasy.in/blog/home-remedies-for-bloating/

Barode, S. (2024c, May 6). Effective home remedies for PCOS. *PharmEasy*. pharmeasy.in/blog/home-remedies-for-pcos/

Barrell, A. (2023, May 30). The best carrier oils for essential oils. Medical News Today. medicalnewstoday.com/articles/321639

Bauer, B. A. (2024, March 27). Herbal treatment for anxiety: Is it effective? Mayo Clinic. mayoclinic.org/diseases-conditions/generalized-anxiety-disorder/expert-answers/herbal-treatment-for-anxiety/faq-20057945

Bedosky, L. (n.d.). Essential oil dos and dont's: Aromatherapy tips for beginners. Everyday Health. everydayhealth.com/wellness/essential-oil-dos-and-donts-aromatherapy-tips-for-beginners/

Bedosky, L. (2022, December 1). 7 herbs and spices that may help boost immunity naturally. Everyday Health.

everydayhealth.com/diet-nutrition/herbs-and-spices-that-may-help-boost-immunity-naturally/

Bedosky, L. (2023, March 3). 4 mood-boosting essential oils to support everyday life challenges. Everyday Health. everydayhealth.com/wellness/mood-boosting-essential-oils-to-support-everyday-life-challenges/

Bell, A. (2023, December 8). 8 home remedies to reduce puffy eyes from crying. Medical News Today. medicalnewstoday.com/articles/how-to-get-rid-of-puffy-eyes-from-crying

Bell, B. (2023, June 23). How to naturally whiten your teeth at home. Healthline. healthline.com/nutrition/whiten-teeth-naturally

Benefits of physical activity. (n.d.). Centers for Disease Control and Prevention. cdc.gov/physicalactivity/basics/pa-health/index.htm

Berry, J. (n.d.). *Dandelion salve recipe {for sore muscles & chapped skin}*. The Nerdy Farm Wife. thenerdyfarmwife.com/dandelion-salve-recipe/

Berry, J. (2024, February 28). 16 natural remedies for eczema. Medical News Today. medicalnewstoday.com/articles/324228

Best herbs for gut health. (2023, August 14). Root Functional Medicine. rootfunctionalmedicine.com/best-herbs-gut-health

Best herbs for UTI treatment: 8 tea recipes. (2024, March). Tua Saúde. tuasaude.com/en/teas-for-uti/

Best home remedies for low blood pressure. (2024, March 21). *PharmEasy*. pharmeasy.in/blog/best-home-remedies-for-low-blood-pressure/

BetterHelp Editorial Team. (2024, April 18). Herbal remedies for mild to moderate depression. BetterHelp. betterhelp.com/advice/depression/the-top-7-best-herbs-for-depression/

Bharat, D. (2021, September 23). Women's health: Ladies, brew these herbal teas to soothe PCOS symptoms. Netmeds. netmeds.com/health-library/post/womens-health-ladies-brew-these-herbal-teas-to-soothe-pcos-symptoms

Black seed - Uses, side effects, and more. (n.d.). WebMD. webmd.com/vitamins/ai/ingredientmono-901/black-seed

Bodhare, A. (2023, November 15). Natural home remedies for ear pain. *PharmEasy*. pharmeasy.in/blog/home-remedies-for-ear-pain/

Bolen, B. (2024, April 15). Supplements and herbs for diarrhea, constipation, and stomach discomfort. Verywell Health. verywellhealth.com/herbs-and-natural-remedies-for-ibs-1944988

Bomgren, L. (2023, September 26). Homemade detox tea recipe: Lemon ginger turmeric tea. Nourish, Move, Love. nourishmovelove.com/lemon-ginger-turmeric-detox-tea/

Boye, K. (2023, January 28). 5 herbs for headaches. Gaia Herbs. gaiaherbs.com/blogs/seeds-of-knowledge/5-herbs-for-headaches

Brandshaw, P. (2023, September 15). [How to make rice water in emergencies]. Be Prepared - Emergency Essentials.

beprepared.com/blogs/articles/how-to-make-rice-water-in-emergencies

Brief history herbal medicine. (n.d.). Herbal Clinic. herbalclinic-swansea.co.uk/herbal-medicine/a-brief-history-of-herbal-medicine/

Bryan, L. (2023, September 17). *Golden milk (turmeric milk).* Downshiftology. downshiftology.com/recipes/turmeric-milk-dairy-free/

Burdock root tea: A soothing and healthful tea recipe. (2023, July 23). The Wild Foodie. wildfoodie.co.uk/post/burdock-root-tea-healthful-beverage

Burgess, L. (2023, October 26). 12 natural ways to relieve pain. Medical News Today. medicalnewstoday.com/articles/324572

Burns. (n.d.). St. Luke's Hospital. stlukes-stl.com/health-content/medicine/33/000021.htm

Byrd, K. (2023, February 2). 8 surprising ingredients that can boost your mood. Taste of Home. tasteofhome.com/collection/ingredients-to-boost-your-mood/

Cadman, B. (2024, January 25). Home remedies for varicose veins. Medical News Today. medicalnewstoday.com/articles/321703#what-are-varicose-veins

Cafasso, J. (2023, February 7). Home remedies for burns. Healthline. healthline.com/health/home-remedies-for-burns

Cafasso, J. (2024, January 30). Home remedies for psoriasis relief. Healthline. healthline.com/health/psoriasis/moderate-to-severe/8-home-remedies-for-psoriasis-do-they-work

Casey, O., & Miller, F. W. (2023, December 1). Autoimmunity has reached epidemic levels. we need urgent action to address it. Scientific American. scientificamerican.com/article/autoimmunity-has-reached-epidemic-levels-we-need-urgent-action-to-address-it/

Casper Editorial Team. (2022, August 15). 4 best herbs for sleep to help you sleep. *Casper*. casper.com/blog/sleep-herbs/

Center for Vein Restoration. (2016, September 6). Home remedies for varicose veins. centerforvein.com/blog/home-remedies-for-varicose-veins

Chang, J. (2024, May 8). 9 natural hair-growth remedies to try at home. GoodRx. goodrx.com/well-being/alternative-treatments/natural-hair-growth-products-remedies

Chappell, S. (2019, December 18). A beginner's guide to making herbal salves and lotions. Healthline. healthline.com/health/diy-herbal-salves

Cherney, K. (2020, May 18). Herbs the word: Help for overactive bladder. Healthline. healthline.com/health/herbs-overactive-bladder

Cherney, K. (2021, June 2). 7 ways to treat an infected wound naturally and when to seek care. Healthline. healthline.com/health/skin/how-to-treat-an-infected-wound-naturally

Cherney, K. (2022, November 15). 9 herbs to fight arthritis pain. Healthline. healthline.com/health/osteoarthritis/herbs-arthritis-pain

Cherney, K. (2023, May 9). What home remedies work for an overactive bladder? Healthline. healthline.com/health/overactive-bladder/home-remedies

Chow, M. (2020, July 3). Everything you need to know about herbal tinctures. Birth Song Botanicals Blog. birthsongbotanicals.com/blogs/birth-song-blog/herbal-tinctures

Christine. (n.d.). *Guest post: How to brew saw palmetto herbal tea.* Just Glowing with Health. justglowingwithhealth.com/guest-posthow-to-brew-saw-palmetto-herbal-tea

Clare, E. (2021, May 7). *Bye-Bye, boils! 10 ways to heal a boil at home.* Greatist. greatist.com/health/home-remedies-for-boils

Coleus root (Coleus forskohlii) 50g. (n.d.). Herbs to Use. herbs-to-use.com/product/coleus-root-50g-coleus-forskohlii/

Comfrey oil and balm recipes. (n.d.). *EarthDance.* earthdancefarms.org/blog/comfrey-oil-and-balm-recipes/

Complementary and alternative medicine. (n.d.). St. Luke's Hospital. stlukes-stl.com/health-content/medicine/33/000157.htm

Complementary and alternative medicine products and their regulation by the Food and Drug Administration. (2006, December). U.S. Food and Drug Administration. fda.gov/regulatory-information/search-fda-guidancedocuments/complementary-and-alternative-medicine-products-and-their-regulation-food-and-drug-administration

Crataeva bark | Crataeva nurvala | Organic. (n.d.). The Apothecary. the-apothecary.co.nz/store/crataeva-bark-crataeva-nurvala-organic/

Cronkleton, E. (2024a, January 9). 10 ways to get rid of bruises. Healthline. healthline.com/health/how-to-get-rid-of-bruises

Cronkleton, E. (2024b, January 17). Home remedies for kidney stones: What works? Healthline. healthline.com/health/kidney-health/home-remedies-for-kidney-stones

Cunha, J. P. (n.d.). Bruises (bruising). eMedicineHealth. emedicinehealth.com/bruises/article_em.htm

Danahy, A. (2019, July 17). 6 powerful teas that fight inflammation. Healthline. healthline.com/nutrition/anti-inflammatory-tea

Danielle. (2015, April 25). *Brahmi: The health benefits and uses of a mind-boosting brain tonic.* Svastha Ayurveda. svasthaayurveda.com/brahmi-the-health-benefits-and-uses-of-a-mind-boosting-brain-tonic/

Davidson, K. (2020, July 8). Bladderwrack: Benefits, uses, and side effects. Healthline. healthline.com/nutrition/bladderwrack-benefits

de la Forêt, R. (2012, November 1). *How to make cayenne salve for herbal pain relief.* LearningHerbs. learningherbs.com/remedies-recipes/herbal-pain-relief/

DeCredico, I. (2022, October 19). *How to make an herbal decoction*. LearningHerbs. learningherbs.com/remedies-recipes/how-to-make-an-herbal-decoction/

Degrandpre, Z. (2023, December 20). How to create a poultice. wikiHow. wikihow.com/Create-a-Poultice

DeKnock, J. (n.d.). *Tranquilizing cat's claw (una de gato) chai tea tonic*. Gourmet Safari. gourmetsafari.com/recipes/cats-claw-una-de-gato-chai-tea/

Delio, M. (2021, March 15). How to make aloe vera juice. Yummy Mummy Kitchen. yummymummykitchen.com/2021/03/aloe-vera-juice-drink.html

DeSoto, L. (2023, January 24). 9 remedies for fast indigestion relief. Verywell Health. verywellhealth.com/indigestion-relief-options-6385942

Dessinger, H. (2022, February 20). *DIY liver love detox support tincture recipe*. Mommypotamus. mommypotamus.com/liver-tincture-recipe/

Deysach, B. (n.d.). Nymph and woodsman wellness: When summer fun hurts: Herbs for twists, sprains, and bone injuries. Nymph and Woodsman. nymphandwoodsman.com/healingmagicblog/when-summer-fun-hurts-herbs-for-twists-springs-and-bone-injuries

Dimuro, C. (2022, February 25). The difference between balms, ointments and salves. Skincare. skincare.com/product-picks/moisturizers/balm-vs-ointment

Discreetlyfit. (2019, March 27). 5 herbs for an overactive bladder. Discreetly Fit. discreetlyfit.com.au/herbs-for-overactive-bladder/

DIY detox tea recipes for radiant skin. (n.d.). *Pure Fiji.* us.purefiji.com/blogs/news/diy-detox-tea-recipes-for-radiant-skin

Do you know the 9 herbs and spices that fight memory loss? (2020, May 26). Amen Clinics. amenclinics.com/blog/do-you-know-the-9-herbs-and-spices-that-fight-memory-loss/

DoctorNDTV. (2018, June 24). World vitiligo day: 10 effective home remedies to treat vitiligo. NDTV. ndtv.com/health/world-vitiligo-day-2018-10-effective-home-remedies-to-treat-vitiligo-1872328

Dresden, D. (2024, April 5). Home remedies for asthma to relieve symptoms naturally. Medical News Today. medicalnewstoday.com/articles/home-remedies-for-asthma

Easy arnica salve for strains, sprains, and bruises. (n.d.). *Golden Vista Farm.* goldenvistafarm.com/blog/easy-arnica-salve-for-sprains-strains-and-bruises

Editor. (2022, March 28). *What are the benefits of herbal medicine?* The Yale Ledger. campuspress.yale.edu/ledger/what-are-the-benefits-of-herbal-medicine/

Editorial Team. (2018, December 21). 4 powerful spiced teas to increase your sex drive. The Health Site. thehealthsite.com/sexual-health/sex/4-powerful-spiced-teas-to-increase-your-sex-drive-634388/

8 effective natural remedies for indigestion. (n.d.). Rennie. rennie.co.uk/tips-advice/tips/indigestion-remedies

8 herbal teas to relieve aches and pains. (n.d.). *NutraTea*. nutratea.co.uk/blogs/8-herbal-teas-to-relieve-aches-and-pains/

8 natural remedies for indigestion. (n.d.). Athreya Herbs. athreyaherbs.com/blogs/news/8-natural-remedies-for-indigestion

8 natural remedies for upset stomach. (2022, November 25). Baptist Health. baptisthealth.com/blog/baptist-health/8-natural-remedies-for-upset-stomach

Elecampane benefits. (n.d.). Indigo Herbs. indigo-herbs.co.uk/natural-health-guide/benefits/elecampane

11 best tea recipes to get rid of nausea. (2023, May). Tua Saúde. tuasaude.com/en/how-to-get-rid-of-nausea/

11 herbs you need to know for immune support. (2022, April 4). Gaia Herbs. gaiaherbs.com/blogs/seeds-of-knowledge/11-herbs-you-need-to-know-for-immune-support

11 natural ways to cure mouth ulcers fast. (2023, April). Tua Saúde. tuasaude.com/en/mouth-ulcers/

Eliminate headaches naturally with herbs. (n.d.). Herbalism Roots. herbalismroots.com/eliminate-headaches-naturally-with-herbs/

Ellis, M. E. (2024, January 24). Natural relief from arthritis pain. Healthline. healthline.com/health/osteoarthritis/arthritis-natural-relief

Eske, J. (2019, March 20). 10 natural remedies for dandruff. Medical News Today. medicalnewstoday.com/articles/324756

Fanous, S. (2024, February 13). 16 natural remedies for mosquito bite relief. Healthline. healthline.com/health/outdoor-health/home-remedies-for-mosquito-bites

Feiereisen, S. (2022, April 13). 21 life-changing detox teas you can make yourself. theFashionSpot. thefashionspot.com/beauty/wellness/687267-detox-teas-recipes/

Fenugreek. (n.d.). PeaceHealth. peacehealth.org/medical-topics/id/hn-2090006

5 herbs and spices for natural detoxification. (2020, December 9). Canyon Ranch. canyonranch.com/well-stated/post/5-herbs-and-spices-for-natural-detoxification/

5 herbs to boost your memory. (n.d.). College of Naturopathic Medicine. naturopathy-uk.com/news/news-cnm-blog/blog/2022/05/23/5-herbs-to-boost-your-memory/

5 herbs to supercharge your immune system. (n.d.). College of Naturopathic Medicine. naturopathy-uk.com/news/blog/2023/04/05/5-herbs-to-supercharge-your-immune-system/

5 home remedies for psoriasis (and other natural treatments). (2023, December). Tua Saúde. tuasaude.com/en/home-remedies-for-psoriasis/

5 natural remedies for poison ivy rashes. (n.d.). Allegheny Kiski Health Foundation. akhealth.org/natural-remedies-for-poison-ivy/

5 of the best exercises you can ever do. (2024, February 20). Harvard Health Publishing. health.harvard.edu/staying-healthy/5-of-the-best-exercises-you-can-ever-do

5 ways to make natural energy drink at home. (2020, August 16). The Times of India. timesofindia.indiatimes.com/life-style/food-news/5-ways-to-make-natural-energy-drink-at-home/photostory/77565993.cms

Fletcher, J. (2023a, November 22). What is an herbal tincture? Recipes and uses. Medical News Today. medicalnewstoday.com/articles/324149

Fletcher, J. (2023b, December 21). 11 natural and home remedies for erectile dysfunction. Medical News Today. medicalnewstoday.com/articles/316291

Fletcher, J. (2023c, December 22). The best herbs to help lower cholesterol. Medical News Today. medicalnewstoday.com/articles/herbs-to-help-lower-cholesterol-quickly

4 ayurvedic detox tea recipes to flush out toxins naturally -. (n.d.). The Art of Living. artofliving.org/in-en/ayurveda/recipes/ayurvedic-tea-to-detox-body

4 easy & accessible dandruff home remedies. (n.d.). Head & Shoulders. headandshoulders.ph/en-ph/scalp/dandruff/dandruff-home-remedies

14 natural remedies for depression. (n.d.). Supernutritious. supernutritious.net/14-natural-remedies-for-depression/

Frothingham, S. (2019, May 24). Which herbs help endometriosis symptoms? Healthline. healthline.com/health/herbs-for-endometriosis

Fulghum, D. (n.d.). Alternative treatments for depression. WebMD. webmd.com/depression/alternative-therapies-depression

Galan, N. (2019a, February 26). 8 herbs and supplements for depression. Medical News Today. medicalnewstoday.com/articles/314421

Galan, N. (2019b, October 4). What are the best natural treatments for PCOS? Medical News Today. medicalnewstoday.com/articles/326560

Galan, N. (2023, October 11). How to get rid of menstrual cramps with 8 home remedies. Medical News Today. medicalnewstoday.com/articles/324484

Gardner, A. (2023a, November 15). Home remedies for diarrhea. Health. health.com/condition/digestive-health/diarrhea-home-remedies

Gardner, A. (2023b, December 31). 8 natural remedies for allergies. Health. health.com/condition/allergy/home-remedies-for-allergies-what-works

Garnsworthy, J. (2018, August 2). 7 herbs that will boost your mood. Studio Pilates. studiopilates.com/7-herbs-that-will-boost-your-mood/

Geerts, J. (2023, June 27). *Making mullein flower ear oil.* Serenity Hill Farmstead. serenityhillfarmstead.com/making-mullein-flower-ear-oil/

Geller, C. A. (n.d.). *Great immune booster recipes for you to enjoy!* French Broad Food Co-Op. frenchbroadfood.coop/great-wellness-recipes-for-you-to-enjoy/

Gentile, R. (2022, October 24). *Eczema relief with natural herbs*. Essendon Natural Health. essendonnaturalhealth.com.au/eczema-relief-with-natural-herbs/

Gibson, B. (2023, April 7). *The best herbal tea blend for energy*. The Homestead Challenge. thehomesteadchallenge.com/the-best-herbal-tea-for-energy/

Gladstar, R. (2021, April 12). Herbal skin care basics: Tools, ingredients, recipes. Mother Earth News. motherearthnews.com/natural-health/herbal-skin-care-zeoz11zhir/

The GlycanAge Team. (n.d.). 14 best natural remedies for muscle pain and inflammation. *GlycanAge*. glycanage.com/glycanhub/blog/health/natural-remedies-for-muscle-pain

Goldman, R. (2023, May 5). 10 effective earache remedies. Healthline. healthline.com/health/11-effective-earache-remedies

Gomez, L. G. (2022, July 15). How to dilute essential oils: A complete guide. *Nikura*. nikura.com/blogs/discover/how-to-dilute-essential-oils-a-complete-guide

Gotter, A. (2023, April 10). Home remedies for boils. Healthline. healthline.com/health/home-remedies-for-boils

Gotu kola tea - The longevity infusion. (n.d.). The Right Tea. therighttea.com/gotu-kola-tea.html

Goyal, A. (2023, January 10). Vitiligo - home remdies to treat vitiligo on body. Lybrate. lybrate.com/topic/suffering-from-vitilgo-how-to-get-rid-of-it/53a02e12b75c32b7476692a48a16feab

Green Goo. (2020, June 11). What is a salve? greengoo.com/blogs/news/what-is-a-salve

Green, A. (2019, July 3). Blessed thistle benefits. Healthline. healthline.com/health/blessed-thistle

Grindelia - Grindelia robusta nut. (n.d.). Living Proof. alivingproof.com/products/grindelia-tea

Groves, M. N. (2021, March 19). *Spring detox herbs & recipes*. Wintergreen Botanicals. wintergreenbotanicals.com/2021/03/19/springdetox/

Groves, M. N. (2023, February 2). *How to make herbal tinctures*. Wintergreen Botanicals. wintergreenbotanicals.com/2020/05/12/tinctures/

A guide to choosing the best herbal solvent. (n.d.). Formula Botanica. formulabotanica.com/herbal-solvent/

Gupta, A. (2020, March 5). 5 herbal drinks that heal and clear your acne from inside out. Vogue India. vogue.in/wellness/content/how-to-get-rid-of-acne-anti-acne-herbal-drinks

Gupta, A. (2021, March 20). Trust these 9 herbs and spices to keep your gut health in check. Healthshots. healthshots.com/healthy-eating/nutrition/trust-these-9-herbs-and-spices-to-keep-your-gut-health-in-check/

Gupta, A. (2022, April 5). Struggling with UTI? Giloy can help. Healthshots. healthshots.com/intimate-health/feminine-hygiene/how-to-treat-uti-at-home-5-herbs-for-uti-relief/

Gupta, A. (2023, October 23). High blood pressure? You can control it with these 5 herbs. Healthshots. healthshots.com/healthy-eating/superfoods/5-herbs-that-can-help-lower-blood-pressure/

Gupta, N. (n.d.). *Nourishing tea recipe for PCOS: Revitalize your morning*. Fitness with Nidhi. fitnesswithnidhi.com/morning-tea-recipe-for-pcos/

Hall, K. (2022, April 21). Natural remedies for depression. Hers. forhers.com/blog/natural-remedies-for-depression

Hareshe, S. (n.d.). natural remedies for hay fever. Pukka Herbs. pukkaherbs.com/uk/en/wellbeing-articles/natural-remedies-for-hay-fever

Harley, J. (2020, January 16). 10 best natural home remedies for IBS. Mindset Health. mindsethealth.com/matter/10-best-natural-home-remedies-for-ibs

Healey, J. (n.d.). *Homemade DIY witch hazel.* Pronounce. pronounceskincare.com/homemade-diy-witch-hazel/

The Healthline Editorial Team. (2023, March 8). 7 natural remedies for high cholesterol. Healthline. healthline.com/health/heart-disease/natural-remedies-cholesterol

The Healthline Editorial Team. (2024, March 27). 6 home remedies and OTC options to help with period cramps. Healthline. healthline.com/health/womens-health/menstrual-cramp-remedies

Healthy diet. (2020, April 29). World Health Organization. who.int/news-room/fact-sheets/detail/healthy-diet

Heck, E. (n.d.). *Top herbs for energy*. Home Herb School. homeherbschool.com/top-herbs-energy/

Heidi. (2020, March 15). Herbal oxymel recipes & benefits. *Mountain Rose Herbs*. blog.mountainroseherbs.com/herbal-oxymels

Heidi. (2022, March 17). A beginner's guide to herbalism. *Mountain Rose Herbs*. blog.mountainroseherbs.com/building-a-herbal-starter-kit

Heirloom Body Care Admin. (2014, July 22). How to make an ointment base. *Heirloom Body Care*. heirloombodycare.com.au/blogs/tutorials/ointment

Hentschel, N. (2016, November 16). *Herbal eyewash for conjunctivitis*. Your Remedy Naturopathy. yourremedy.com.au/herbal-eyewash-for-conjunctivitis/

Herb-drug interactions. (2021, July). National Center for Complementary and Integrative Health. nccih.nih.gov/health/providers/digest/herb-drug-interactions

Herbal Academy. (2015, January 19). 3 herbal recipes to boost your energy. theherbalacademy.com/blog/3-herbal-recipes-to-boost-your-energy/

Herbal Academy. (2019a, August 22). The best places to purchase herbs and supplies world-wide. theherbalacademy.com/blog/purchase-herbs-and-supplies-world-wide/

Herbal Academy. (2019b, September 6). Our favorite herbs to help you get your study on (plus, a DIY memory tonic tea recipe!). theherbalacademy.com/blog/favorite-study-herbs/

Herbal extracts – Health benefits & more. (2022, September 5). Arjuna Natural. arjunanatural.com/herbal-extracts-health-benefits/

Herbal Knowledge. (2023, January 17). 6 herbs for detoxifying. Berkeley Herbal Center. berkeleyherbalcenter.org/detox-herbs/

Herbal medicine. (n.d.-a). Better Health Channel. betterhealth.vic.gov.au/health/ConditionsAndTreatments/herbal-medicine

Herbal medicine. (n.d.-b). John Hopkins Medicine. hopkinsmedicine.org/health/wellness-and-prevention/herbal-medicine

Herbal remedies. (n.d.). Cancer Research UK. cancerresearchuk.org/about-cancer/coping/mental-health-cancer/how-cancer-make-you-feel/depression/treating-depression/herbal-remedies

Herbal remedies and complementary medicines for menopause symptoms. (n.d.). National Health Service. nhs.uk/medicines/hormone-replacement-therapy-hrt/alternatives-to-hormone-replacement-therapy-hrt/herbal-remedies-and-complementary-medicines-for-menopause-symptoms/

Herbal remedies to improve mental health. (n.d.). Elevate Psychiatry. elevatepsychiatry.com/herbal-remedies-to-improve-mental-health/

Herbal tea: A warm cup of herbs to keep PCOS away. (2019, April 2). Conquer PCOS. conquerpcos.org/herbal-tea/

Herbs and spices for heart health. (2020, July 14). *Mercy Health.* blog.mercy.com/herbs-spices-heart-health/

Herbs for hair: The top 5 choices for healthy hair. (2024, March 27). Tofillo. tofillo.com/en/herbs-for-hair-the-top-5-choices-for-healthy-hair/

Herbs for heart health. (2023, January 16). Guthrie. guthrie.org/blog/herbs-heart-health

Herbs for mental and emotional health. (n.d.). *Herbs & Owls.* herbsandowls.com/herbal-medicine-blog/herbs-for-mental-and-emotional-health

Herbs for natural detox. (2019, December 26). Traditional Medicinals. traditionalmedicinals.com/blogs/ppj/herbs-for-natural-detox

Hersh, E. (2024, March 27). 12 healthy sleep hygiene tips. Healthline. healthline.com/health/sleep-hygiene

Higuera, V. (2023, May 15). How to treat indigestion at home. Healthline. healthline.com/health/home-remedies-for-indigestion

Hill, A. (2020, September 30). 10 herbs and supplements for menopause. Healthline. healthline.com/nutrition/menopause-herbs

Hill, A. (2023, February 14). 8 herbs and natural supplements for utis. Healthline. healthline.com/nutrition/herbs-for-uti

Hoffmaster, D. (2023, June 22). How to make your own herbal teas. Treehugger. treehugger.com/how-to-make-your-own-herbal-tea-recipes-and-instructions-5194393

Holland, K., & The Healthline Editorial. (2022, September 30). "Herbal viagra" and herbs to treat erectile dysfunction: Do they work? Healthline. healthline.com/health/erectile-dysfunction/herbs

Home remedies for ED: 6 natural recipes with herbs. (2023, October). Tua Saúde. tuasaude.com/en/home-remedies-for-ed/

Home remedies for pink eye (conjunctivitis). (2022, May 16). MyVision.org. myvision.org/eye-conditions/pink-eye-home-remedies/

Home remedies to bring down your cholesterol naturally. (2019, February 14). The Times of India. timesofindia.indiatimes.com/life-style/food-news/home-remedies-to-bring-down-your-cholesterol-naturally/photostory/67988685.cms

How herbs can soothe headaches and migraines. (n.d.). *Zen Maitri*. zenmaitri.com/blogs/news/how-herbs-can-soothe-headaches-and-migraines

How to brew the perfect cup of neem tea. (2015, June 2). Neem Tree Farms. neemtreefarms.com/how-to-brew-the-perfect-cup-of-neem-tea/

How to get rid of hay fever with 5 pollen-proof remedies. (n.d.). Cushelle. cushelle.com/hygiene-and-care/household-remedies/5-natural-remedies-for-hay-fever/

How to get rid of pink eye fast. (2021, January 7). Monitor. monitor.co.ug/uganda/magazines/healthy-living/how-to-get-rid-of-pink-eye-fast-1758646

How to improve your mental wellbeing. (2023, August). Mind. mind.org.uk/information-support/tips-for-everyday-living/wellbeing/

How to make a decoction. (2020, January 20). wikiHow. wikihow.com/Make-a-Decoction

How to make a herbal steam inhalation. (2023, April 8). Herbal Reality. herbalreality.com/herbalism/home-herbalism/making-medicines/how-to-make-herbal-steam-inhalation/

How to make a simple healing salve recipe. (n.d.). The Old Walsh Farm. theoldwalshfarm.com/bee-gyms-and-honey-hand-salve/

How to make buchu tea. (2023, October 24). BuchuVida. buchuvida.com/blog/how-to-make-buchu-tea

How to make herbal balms: A beginner's guide & easy recipe. (2020, September 18). Gaia Herbs. gaiaherbs.com/blogs/seeds-of-knowledge/how-to-make-herbal-balms-a-beginners-guide-and-easy-recipe

How to make homemade echinacea tea. (n.d.). *Sencha*. senchateabar.com/blogs/blog/how-to-make-echinacea-tea

How to make reishi tea. (2020, October 23). *Cascadia Mushrooms*. cascadiamushrooms.com/blogs/recipes/how-to-make-reishi-tea

Huizen, J. (2023, November 30). 12 home remedies for stomach pain. Medical News Today. medicalnewstoday.com/articles/322047

Huizen, J. (2024a, February 14). 16 home remedies to get rid of acne. Medical News Today. medicalnewstoday.com/articles/322455

Huizen, J. (2024b, May 3). Home remedies for boils. Medical News Today. medicalnewstoday.com/articles/319939

Hutchison, M. (2018, February 1). Must-have tools for herbalists. *Mountain Rose Herbs*. blog.mountainroseherbs.com/tools-for-herbalists

Iftikhar, N. (2023, July 11). 10 natural remedies for flu symptoms. Healthline. healthline.com/health/natural-flu-remedies

Iliades, C. (n.d.). 14 herbs and spices for rheumatoid arthritis symptom relief. Everyday Health. everydayhealth.com/rheumatoid-arthritis/diet/six-herbs-and-spices-for-rheumatoid-arthritis/

Institute for Natural Medicine Staff. (2023, November 17). *How naturopathic doctors treat endometriosis*. Institute for Natural Medicine. naturemed.org/how-do-naturopathic-doctors-treat-endometriosis/

Irene. (2019, August 13). How to make herb-infused oils for culinary & body care use. *Mountain Rose Herbs*. blog.mountainroseherbs.com/making-herbal-oils

Janis. (2024a, January 15). *How to get rid of bags under your eyes*. Health Nile. healthnile.com/how-to-get-rid-of-bags-under-your-eyes/?utm_source=google&utm_medium=CjwKCAjwl4yyBhAgEiwADSEjeLjM-bp-YnKyvT7niXXwsUViadqrxGEh8v3WwDUqvHu9emobN2QtixoCJzgQAvD_BwE&cuid=CjwKCAjwl4yyBhAgEiwADSEjeLjM-bp-YnKyvT7niXXwsUViadqrxGEh8v3WwDUqvHu9emobN2QtixoCJzgQAvD_BwE&gad_source=1&gclid=CjwKCAjwl4yyBhAgEiwADSEjeLjM-bp-

YnKyvT7niXXwsUViadqrxGEh8v3WwDUqvHu9em0bN2QtixoCJzgQAvD_BwE

Janis. (2024b, January 16). *Sore throat: 7 natural remedies (that actually work)*. HealthNile. healthnile.com/sore-throat-7-natural-remedies-that-actually-work/

Janis. (2024c, January 19). *How to get rid of a cough*. HealthNile. healthnile.com/how-to-get-rid-of-a-cough/

Janis. (2024d, January 22). *How to relieve sinus pressure*. HealthNile. healthnile.com/how-to-relieve-sinus-pressure/

Jerajani, D. (2024, January 9). 7 powerful home remedies for acne! *PharmEasy*. pharmeasy.in/blog/7-powerful-home-remedies-for-acne/

Jhon, J. (2023, December). 10 best herbs for energy: How to fight general fatigue. Life Extension. lifeextension.com/wellness/herbs-spices/herbs-for-energy

Johnson, J. (2023, November 24). 8 herbal teas for constipation. Medical News Today. medicalnewstoday.com/articles/322624

Joint pain salve. (n.d.). Mary Tylor Naturals. marytylor.com/recipe/joint-pain-salve

Jones, H. (2023, December 29). 7 home remedies for ear infections. Verywell Health. verywellhealth.com/home-remedies-ear-infections-5180182

Jovinally, J. (2024, February 2). Cold and flu home remedies. Healthline. healthline.com/health/cold-flu/home-remedies

Joybilee Farm. (n.d.). *DIY headache salve from your garden*. joybileefarm.com/headache-salve/?customize_changeset_uuid=

Kamble, B. (2023, May 30). Herbs for mental and emotional wellbeing. *Herbal Apothecary UK*. herbalapothecaryuk.com/blogs/news/herbs-for-mental-and-emotional-wellbeing

Kandola, A. (2023, October 13). How to treat diarrhea at home. Medical News Today. medicalnewstoday.com/articles/324424

Karen, S. (2019, January 13). *Herbal remedies notebook*. No Fuss Natural. nofussnatural.com/herbal-remedies-notebook/

Kendle. (2018, September 14). How to make herbal infusions & decoctions for wellness support. *Mountain Rose Herbs*. blog.mountainroseherbs.com/herbal-infusions-and-decoctions

Khan, J. (2023, August 4). Essential oils for vitiligo - skin treatment for white patches. VedaOils. vedaoils.com/blogs/essentialoils/essential-oils-for-vitiligo

Kharbanda, N. (2020, December 16). Here are 10 natural remedies to heal minor wounds. Onlymyhealth. onlymyhealth.com/here-are-10-natural-remedies-to-heal-minor-wounds-1608097698

Kiefer, D. (2018, August 20). Herbs and supplements for acid reflux (GERD). Healthline. healthline.com/health/gerd-herbs-supplements

kim. (2010, July 20). Horny goats weed decoction. Real Foods. realfoods.co.uk/recipe/horny-goats-weed-decoction

Klein, E., & McDonnell, K. (2023, February 14). How to get rid of acne: 14 home remedies for pimples. Healthline. healthline.com/nutrition/13-acne-remedies

Kotsiris, K. (2023, February 8). Marjoram tea. The Spruce Eats. thespruceeats.com/greek-marjoram-tea-1705055

Krans, B. (2023, November 16). 8 ways to treat sunburn at home. Healthline. healthline.com/health/sunburn

Kukreja, K. (n.d.). 16 simple ways to get white teeth overnight. Stylecraze. stylecraze.com/articles/simple-ways-to-get-white-teeth-overnight/?sem_campaign=PMAXDynRemedies_SouthAfrica&gad_source=1&gclid=CjwKCAjwl4yyBhAgEiwADSEjeOYn-uKBB3R5-kueOsXP5dVGZxBZXEQ84BIH1hAWbcLMiIZhicvUoxoCRVkQAvD_BwE

Kukreja, K. (2023, November 14). How to stop coughing – 26 home remedies that can help. StyleCraze. stylecraze.com/articles/effective-home-remedies-to-get-rid-of-cough/

La Forge, T. (2019, June 3). Drink "moon milk" with ashwagandha at night to lower stress, improve sleep. Healthline. healthline.com/health/food-nutrition/moon-milk-ashwagandha

La Forge, T. (2020, April 23). 8 herbs, spices, and sweeteners that combine to activate your immune system. Healthline. healthline.com/health/food-nutrition/immune-system-bitters-recipe

Lawler, M. (n.d.). Ear infection home remedies. Everyday Health. everydayhealth.com/ear-infection/home-remedies/

Leonard, J. (2017, April 24). Natural remedies for an overactive bladder. Medical News Today. medicalnewstoday.com/articles/317091

Lewittes, E. (2022, July 5). 10 best herbs for eczema to repair skin inflammation. Zensa Skin Care. zensaskincare.com/blogs/news/herbs-for-eczema-treatment

Licorice. (n.d.). Mount Sinai. mountsinai.org/health-library/herb/licorice

Lockett, E. (2023, February 8). 9 ways to naturally clear up your congestion. Healthline. healthline.com/health/natural-decongestant

Lyon, L. (n.d.). Herb article peony. Rebecca's Herbal Apothecary. rebeccasherbs.com/pages/herb-article-br-peony.html

Macfarlane, S. (2021a, September 3). The 5 most powerful mood boosting herbs. *Wild Dispensary*. wilddispensary.co.nz/blogs/news/mood-boosting-herbs

Macfarlane, S. (2021b, October 8). 8 incredible herbs to help with sleep. *Wild Dispensary*. wilddispensary.co.nz/blogs/news/herbs-to-help-with-sleep

Make: Herbal infused oils. (n.d.). Handmade Apothecary. handmadeapothecary.co.uk/infused-oils-intro

Malka, T. (2021, December 21). *Herbs and plants for high blood pressure*. K Health. khealth.com/learn/hypertension/herbs-for-high-blood-pressure/

Marie. (2015, August 27). Lady cramp salve. Humblebee & Me. humblebeeandme.com/lady-cramp-salve/

Marketing. (2022, March 8). *A whole body approach to treatment: Mind, body, and spirit.* Dream Recovery. dreamrecovery.com/a-whole-body-approach-to-treatment-mind-body-and-spirit/

Mars, B. (n.d.). *Herbs for mental and emotional health [Fact sheet].* American Herbalists Guild. americanherbalistsguild.com/sites/default/files/Proceedings/mars_brigitte_-_herbs_for_mental_and_emotional_health.pdf

May, B. (2023, June 13). 15 effective options for treating earache. Medical News Today. medicalnewstoday.com/articles/312634

Mayo Clinic Staff. (2024, January 26). Bags under eyes. Mayo Clinic. mayoclinic.org/diseases-conditions/bags-under-eyes/diagnosis-treatment/drc-20369931

McCulloch, M., & Ajmera, R. (2023, April 4). 8 herbal teas to help reduce bloating. Healthline. healthline.com/nutrition/tea-for-bloating

McDermott, A. (2017, March 22). Can you use herbs to treat acne? Healthline. healthline.com/health/beauty-skin-care/herbs-for-acne

McDermott, A. (2018a, June 15). 19 herbal remedies for hair growth. Healthline. healthline.com/health/herbs-for-hair-growth

McDermott, A. (2018b, October 5). 5 herbal remedies for constipation. Healthline. healthline.com/health/digestive-health/herbal-remedies-for-constipation

McDermott, A. (2024a, January 19). Ways to get rid of canker sores (aphthous ulcer). Healthline. healthline.com/health/dental-and-oral-health/how-to-get-rid-of-canker-sores

McDermott, A. (2024b, February 1). How to stop throwing up and ways to find nausea relief. Healthline. healthline.com/health/how-to-stop-vomiting-remedies

McIntosh, J. (2023, December 21). Fifteen benefits of drinking water. Medical News Today. medicalnewstoday.com/articles/290814

Menopause. (n.d.). Cleveland Clinic. my.clevelandclinic.org/health/diseases/21841-menopause

Meyer, A. (2023, May 24). The 6 best spices to fight gut inflammation, according to gastroenterologists. EatingWell. eatingwell.com/article/8047957/best-spices-for-gut-inflammation/

Miller, K. (n.d.). Erectile dysfunction treatment. WebMD. webmd.com/erectile-dysfunction/erectile-dysfunction-treatment

Momaya, A. (2022, March 8). Giloy: Healthy recipes. HealthifyMe. healthifyme.com/blog/giloy-healthy-recipes/

Mondia whitei (white ginger) tea. (n.d.). Smoky Hazel. smokyhazelspice.com/products/mondia-whitei-white-ginger-tea

Moses, A. (2023, September 11). 19 surprisingly effective home remedies for insect bites & stings. Chemist4U. chemist-4-u.com/guides/travel/home-remedies-for-insect-bites-and-stings/

Mouth ulcers: 5 amazing kitchen remedies to heal canker sores. (2022, September 18). Netmeds.com. netmeds.com/health-library/post/mouth-ulcers-5-amazing-kitchen-remedies-to-heal-canker-sores

Murphy, S., & Sharon, A. (2023, May 10). 14 natural ways to help treat severe asthma. Healthline. healthline.com/health/severe-asthma/natural-remedies

Nall, R. (2018, April 21). Can essential oils reduce varicose veins? Medical News Today. medicalnewstoday.com/articles/321562

Natural mouth ulcer remedies. (2023, October 25). Colgate. colgate.com/en-gb/oral-health/gastrointestinal-disorders/ways-to-get-rid-of-mouth-ulcers-naturally

Natural remedies for hot flashes. (n.d.). The North American Menopause Society. menopause.org/for-women/menopauseflashes/menopause-symptoms-and-treatments/natural-remedies-for-hot-flashes

Natural remedies for IBS. (n.d.). London Gastroenterology Centre. gastrolondon.co.uk/irritable-bowel-syndrome/natural-remedies-for-ibs/

Natural remedies for menstrual cramps: 12 teas to try. (2022, November). Tua Saúde. tuasaude.com/en/natural-remedies-for-menstrual-cramps/

Natural remedies for soothing a persistent cough. (2023, July 18). Dis-Chem. dischem.co.za/articles/post/natural-remedies-for-soothing-a-persistent-cough?

NDTV Food. (2018, August 21). *7 effective home remedies for low blood pressure*. food.ndtv.com/health/home-remedies-for-low-blood-pressure-1287697

Nice, S. (2023, August 10). The very best essential oils for uplifting your mood and boosting happiness. *NEOM Wellbeing UK*. neomwellbeing.com/blogs/mood/best-essential-oils-for-uplifting-mood-and-boosting-happiness

9 herbs to help support a healthy and happy heart. (2023, April 4). Gaia Herbs. gaiaherbs.com/blogs/seeds-of-knowledge/herbs-to-help-support-a-healthy-and-happy-heart

Nourish'd. (2018, December 18). 8 natural remedies to cure hay fever fast. *Nourish'd Café*. nourishd.co.za/blogs/news/8-natural-remedies-to-cure-hay-fever-fast

Noveille, A. (2019, January 22). The herbal tools I use the most in my home apothecary. *Indie Herbalist*. blog.indieherbalist.com/herbal-tools-of-the-trade/

Noveille, A. (2023, October 16). *How to make eleuthero tea*. Teacup Alchemy. teacupalchemy.com/eleuthero-tea/

O'Brien, K. (2020, October 20). 8 all-natural ways to kick your immune system into fight mode this flu season. *Bee Potion*. beepotion.co.uk/blogs/news/8-all-natural-ways-boost-your-immune-system-this-winter

Oliveira, D. (2022, May 19). 13 home remedies for high blood pressure. Tua Saúde. tuasaude.com/en/natural-remedies-for-high-blood-pressure/

Oliver, K. (2015, December 23). *Honey & chamomile home remedy for pink eye*. Dr. Axe. draxe.com/beauty/home-remedy-for-pink-eye/

Pal, A. (2024, March 22). Simple home remedies for varicose veins. *PharmEasy*. pharmeasy.in/blog/simple-home-remedies-for-varicose-veins/

Panoff, L. (2023, January 11). 11 best herbs and supplements for high blood pressure. Verywell Health. verywellhealth.com/herbs-and-supplements-to-naturally-lower-blood-pressure-6466120

Patricia. (2021, March 8). 5 natural remedies for seasonal allergies. Detroit Sinus Center. detroitsinuscenter.com/blog/sinus-doctor-detroit/5-natural-remedies-seasonal-allergies/

Patricia. (2023, January 27). Home remedies that can help with allergies. Detroit Sinus Center. detroitsinuscenter.com/allergies/home-remedies-can-help-allergies/

Pedersen, T. (2023, July 5). 3 easy homemade creams for eczema relief. Healthline. healthline.com/health/eczema/homemade-cream-for-eczema

Peer, A. (2020, November 6). Natural cold and flu remedies from around the world. World Vision. worldvision.org/health-news-stories/natural-cold-flu-remedies-world

Penrod, S. (n.d.). *Sweet dreams tea.* Urban Cowgirl. urbancowgirllife.com/sweet-dreams-tea/

Perry, J. (2023a, May 24). *Dong quai tea: Benefits, side effects, and how to make it.* Chinese Teas 101. chineseteas101.com/dong-quai-tea-benefits-side-effects/

Perry, J. (2023b, May 24). *Evening primrose tea: Benefits, side effects, and how to make it.* Chinese Teas 101. chineseteas101.com/evening-primrose-tea-benefits-side-effects/

Petrarca, M. (2022, October 3). How to do a skin-care patch test — And why it matters. Everyday Health. everydayhealth.com/skin-beauty/how-to-do-a-skin-care-patch-test/

Petre, A. (2020, June 18). Goldenseal: Benefits, dosage, side effects, and more. Healthline. healthline.com/health/goldenseal-cure-for-everything

Petre, A. (2023, June 12). Natural ways to get rid of nausea, plus tips. Healthline. healthline.com/nutrition/nausea-remedies

PlacideO. (2023, March 9). *How to make juniper berry tea.* Steeped Street. steepedstreet.com/how-to-make-juniper-berry-tea/

Poslusny, C. (2022, September 16). 10 science-backed natural remedies for congestion. *Molekule.* molekule.com/blogs/all/10-science-backed-natural-remedies-for-congestion

Pristyn Care Team. (2023, October 19). 20 home remedies for kidney stones. Pristyn Care. pristyncare.com/blog/home-remedies-for-kidney-stones/

Purwar, K. (2023, June 16). Dil se indian: Herbal tea recipe using cumin and coriander seeds to manage PCOS. Her Zindagi. herzindagi.com/advice/herbal-tea-recipe-to-manage-pcos-article-234489

Quinn, J. (2023, May 15). 11 herbs for better sleep. HUM Nutrition. humnutrition.com/blog/11-herbs-for-better-sleep/

Recipe: Soothing osteoarthritis tea. (n.d.). Liebscher & Bracht. liebscher-bracht.com/en/nutrition/recipes/osteoarthritis-tea/

Reddy, M. R. (2021, June 30). 5 reasons to be cautious when considering herbal remedies. Penn Medicine Lancaster General Health. lancastergeneralhealth.org/health-hub-home/2021/june/5-reasons-to-be-cautious-when-considering-herbal-remedies

Relief in sight: Home remedies for pink eye. (2023, November 3). Beaufort Memorial. bmhsc.org/blog/relief-in-sight-home-remedies-for-pink-eye

Remy. (2024, March 14). How to make corn silk tea (plus health benefits!). *Veggiekins*. veggiekinsblog.com/2022/07/11/corn-silk-tea/

Reproductive system. (n.d.). National Cancer Institute. cancer.gov/publications/dictionaries/cancer-terms/def/reproductive-system

Richards, L. (2023, February 9). 9 herbs for anxiety. Medical News Today. medicalnewstoday.com/articles/herbs-for-anxiety

Richards, S. (n.d.). *The health highs of Misty Mountain*. Christian Today. christiantoday.com.au/news/the-health-highs-of-misty-mountain.html

Ridaeus, D. (2023, February 22). Floral and herbal remedies – Gems from the garden of natural mental health. Alternative to Meds. alternativetomeds.com/blog/floral-herbal-remedies/

Robinson, K. (2022, April 28). 10 natural ways to lower your cholesterol. GoodRx. goodrx.com/conditions/high-cholesterol/10-natural-ways-to-lower-your-cholesterol

Rose Wellness. (2023, September 28). *15 natural remedies for constipation.* rosewellness.com/natural-remedies-for-constipation/

Rose, C. (2023, April 7). April 2023 DIY recipe: Detoxifying burdock root tincture. *Organic Alcohol Co.* oacinsider.organicalcohol.com/blog/diy-recipes-detoxifying-burdock-root-tincture

Rowden, A. (2024, January 18). 6 ways to make a wound heal faster. Medical News Today. medicalnewstoday.com/articles/how-to-make-a-wound-heal-faster#should-wounds-be-covered

Sacks, R. (2024, March 5). Erection tea: Does it work for ED? hims. hims.com/blog/erection-tea

Santos-Longhurst, A. (2019a, May 17). What is a poultice and how can I use it to relieve inflammation? Healthline. healthline.com/health/poultice

Santos-Longhurst, A. (2019b, June 18). How to get smooth skin through healthy living, OTC products and treatments. Healthline. healthline.com/health/smooth-skin

saranyabalan7. (2019, September 26). *How to make a herbal skullcap chamomile tea?* Vriksha Homeware. vrikshahomeware.com/how-to-make-a-herbal-tea-for-vibrant-health/

Sarnataro, B. R. (n.d.). 7 most effective exercises. WebMD. webmd.com/fitness-exercise/features/7-most-effective-exercises

Schaefer, A., & Weiss, K. (2021, December 16). 10 natural remedies for IBS. Healthline.

healthline.com/health/irritable-bowel-syndrome/5-natural-products-for-ibs

Schisandra: The berry that does it all. (2015, January 21). Flowerfolk Herbal Apothecary. flowerfolkherbs.com/articles/schisandra-the-berry-that-does-it-all

Schofield, K. (2023, February 4). 7 natural remedies for your upset stomach. Healthline. healthline.com/health/digestive-health/natural-upset-stomach-remedies

Segoviano, A. (2023, October 13). 8 energizing herbal teas that will wake you right up—Without a speck of caffeine. Well+Good. wellandgood.com/energizing-herbal-teas/

Semenovskaya, Z. (n.d.). *Home remedies for boils*. K Health. khealth.com/learn/skin/home-remedies-for-boils/

7 natural remedies to soothe sunburnt skin. (n.d.). *SunDoctors*. sundoctors.com.au/blog/natural-remedies-to-soothe-sunburnt-skin/

Shane, C. (2023, May 10). *Herbal remedies for poison ivy*. Blue Ridge School of Herbal Medicine. blueridgeschool.org/herbal-remedies-for-poison-ivy/

Sharma, P. (2023, November 10). Hypotension: 5 best home remedies to maintain blood pressure. Netmeds. netmeds.com/health-library/post/hypotension-5-best-home-remedies-to-maintain-blood-pressure

Shatavari root tea (asparagus root) - Organic. (n.d.). Zee Tea Organic. zeetea.com.au/products/shatavari-root-tea-organic

Sherrell, Z. (2023, October 5). 15 home remedies for migraine relief and prevention. Medical News Today. medicalnewstoday.com/articles/322814

Shoemaker, S. (2020, October 1). 15 brain-boosting juices and beverages. Healthline. healthline.com/nutrition/juice-for-brain

Sierralupe, S. (n.d.-a). *Antibiotic salve recipe*. The Practical Herbalist. thepracticalherbalist.com/healthy-recipes/herbal-remedies/antibiotic-salve/

Sierralupe, S. (n.d.-b). *Sprained ankle: Herbal first aid*. The Practical Herbalist. thepracticalherbalist.com/advanced-herbalism/first-aid/herbal-first-aid-sprained-ankle/

Singh, M. (2023, May 1). Gut: 5 herbs & spices to reduce bloating. NDTV. ndtv.com/health/gut-5-herbs-spices-to-reduce-bloating-3995537

Singh, S. (2022, May 25). Say goodbye to high cholesterol: Home remedies and lifestyle changes that work. Truemeds. truemeds.in/blog/home-remedies-to-reduce-cholesterol

SingleCare Team. (2023, April 11). 20 home remedies for ear infections. The Checkup. singlecare.com/blog/home-remedies-for-ear-infection/

Sissons, B. (2023, May 17). The 9 best herbs for joint pain. Medical News Today. medicalnewstoday.com/articles/325760

Sissons, C. (2023, January 6). What home remedies can relieve sinus pressure? Medical News Today. medicalnewstoday.com/articles/321322

6 best herbs for UTI treatment. (n.d.). *NutraTea*. nutratea.co.uk/blogs/herbs-for-uti-treatment/

6 herbs that boost energy and increase concentration. (2020, October 7). The Times of India. timesofindia.indiatimes.com/life-style/food-news/6-herbs-that-boost-energy-and-increase-concentration/photostory/78532882.cms

6 tips: How herbs can interact with medicines. (n.d.). National Center for Complementary and Integrative Health. nccih.nih.gov/health/tips/tips-how-herbs-can-interact-with-medicines

6 ways to get rid of bruises (home care & when to see a doctor). (n.d.). Tua Saúde. tuasaude.com/en/how-to-get-rid-of-bruises/

Sowa, A. (2023, April 6). 48 natural remedies to treat symptoms of PCOS. *SoWell Health.* getsowell.com/blogs/pcos/48-natural-remedies-to-treat-symptoms-of-pcos

Spritzler, F. (2024, February 20). 15 natural remedies for a sore throat. Medical News Today. medicalnewstoday.com/articles/318631

Stewart, G. (2023, June 30). How to use herbs for tea - Fresh or dried. Getty Stewart. gettystewart.com/how-to-use-herbs-for-tea/

Stewart, S. (n.d.). Devils claw salve. Just A Pinch Recipes. justapinch.com/recipes/non-edible/other-non-edible/devils-claw-salve.html

Stickler, T. (2023, November 16). Migraine herbal home remedies from around the world. Healthline. healthline.com/health/migraine-herbal-home-remedies-from-around-the-world

Stop the itch: Home remedies to help manage eczema. (n.d.). Cleveland Clinic. health.clevelandclinic.org/home-remedies-for-eczema

Story , C. M., Gotter, A., & Seladi-Schulman, J. (2024, January 8). Sore throat remedies that work (and what not to do). Healthline. healthline.com/health/cold-flu/sore-throat-natural-remedies

Streit, L. (2020, June 4). Oak bark: Benefits, dosage, side effects, and more. Healthline. healthline.com/nutrition/oak-bark

Suni, E. (2024, March 4). Mastering sleep hygiene: Your path to quality sleep. Sleep Foundation. sleepfoundation.org/sleep-hygiene

Swan, J. S. P. (2022, January 24). 9 super herbs and spices for gut health. Parkway East Hospital. parkwayeast.com.sg/health-plus/article/super-herbs-spices

Synergy. (n.d.). Herbal Clinic. herbalclinic-swansea.co.uk/herbal-medicine/synergy/

Tague, A. (n.d.). 4 natural remedies for wounds and scrapes. Tom's of Maine. tomsofmaine.com/good-matters/healthy-feeling/4-natural-remedies-for-wounds-and-scrapes

Talerico, D. (2023, February 22). *How to make salve or balms 101: Simple flexible recipe.* Homestead and Chill. homesteadandchill.com/make-salve-or-balms-recipe-101/

Tea for bloating: 10 natural recipes to relieve gas. (2023, July). Tua Saúde. tuasaude.com/en/tea-for-bloating/

Tea time: Our favorite immune-boosting teas and tonics. (2020, November 27). Tuesday Foods. tuesdayfoods.co/recipes-

and-
resources/2020/11/27/4pznwfvdghmvl8yrut346qsjpksv4y

Tekurio, K. (2023, April 26). *Easy herbal period pain relief cream recipe*. Kateable. kateable.com/easy-herbal-period-pain-relief-cream-recipe/

10 best home remedies for UTI treatment: Teas, juices & more. (2022, December). Tua Saúde. tuasaude.com/en/home-remedies-for-uti/

10 effective home remedies to cure boils. (n.d.). Anveya. anveya.com/blogs/top-tips/10-effective-home-remedies-to-cure-boils

10 herbs for sleep and sleep-related struggles. (n.d.). ZzzQuil. zzzquil.com/en-us/article/herbs-for-sleep-struggles

10 herbs to avoid if you have a heart condition. (n.d.). Supernutritious. supernutritious.net/10-herbs-to-avoid-if-you-have-a-heart-condition/

10 home remedies for a cough. (n.d.). Supernutritious. supernutritious.net/10-home-remedies-for-a-cough/

10 home remedies for a sore throat. (n.d.). Supernutritious. supernutritious.net/10-home-remedies-for-a-sore-throat-2/

10 home remedies for bruises. (n.d.). Supernutritious. supernutritious.net/10-home-remedies-for-bruises/

10 home remedies for headaches. (n.d.). Supernutritious. supernutritious.net/10-home-remedies-for-headaches/

10 home remedies for high cholesterol. (n.d.). Supernutritious. supernutritious.net/10-home-remedies-for-high-cholesterol/

10 home remedies for pink eye. (n.d.). Supernutritious. supernutritious.net/10-home-remedies-for-pink-eye/

10 home remedies for sunburn. (n.d.). Supernutritious. supernutritious.net/10-home-remedies-for-sunburn/

10 natural remedies for poison ivy. (n.d.). Supernutritious. supernutritious.net/10-natural-remedies-for-poison-ivy/

10 plants to help support immune function. (n.d.). *Goldthread*. drinkgoldthread.com/blogs/plants-with-benefits/10-plants-to-help-support-immune-function

10 ways to remove varicose veins. (n.d.). Supernutritious. supernutritious.net/10-ways-to-remove-varicose-veins/

The best home remedy for teeth whitening that works. (n.d.). Colgate. Retrieved May 14, 2024, from colgate.com/en-za/oral-health/teeth-whitening/the-best-home-remedy-for-teeth-whitening?gad_source=1&gclid=CjwKCAjwl4yyBhAgEiwADSEjeIWhcV-bZ_-gYgrHOcYuSqijmK8FiAFgwE__fjrIuDLuq-vtPrJYWRoCxekQAvD_BwE&gclsrc=aw.ds

Theobald, M. (2023, December 26). Best natural ingredients for psoriasis. Everyday Health. everydayhealth.com/psoriasis/treatment/natural-ingredients-psoriasis/

Three recipes to help ease symptoms of endometriosis. (n.d.). Institute for Optimum Nutrition. ion.ac.uk/news/three-recipes-to-help-ease-symptoms-of-endometriosis

TimesofIndia.com. (2023, May 16). *10 home remedies for a super soft skin*. The Times of India. timesofindia.indiatimes.com/life-style/beauty/10-home-remedies-for-a-super-soft-skin/articleshow/100244293.cms

Top 7 home remedies for kidney stones. (2023, July). Tua Saúde. tuasaude.com/en/home-remedies-for-kidney-stones/

Toshi, N. (2024a, April 1). *10 ways to clear stuffy nose with home remedies*. PharmEasy. pharmeasy.in/blog/10-ways-to-clear-stuffy-nose-with-home-remedies/

Toshi, N. (2024b, May 3). 12 natural remedies for mouth ulcers. *PharmEasy*. pharmeasy.in/blog/12-natural-remedies-to-cure-mouth-ulcers/

Toshi, N. (2024c, May 3). 15 home remedies to cure dandruff naturally. *PharmEasy*. pharmeasy.in/blog/15-home-remedies-to-cure-dandruff-naturally/

Toshi, N. (2024d, May 3). 16 simple home remedies for glowing skin! *PharmEasy*. pharmeasy.in/blog/simple-home-remedies-for-glowing-skin/

Tourles, S. (2013, October 14). Topical herbal pain relief salve. Stephanie Tourles. stephanietourles.com/post/topical-herbal-pain-relief-salve

Tribulus terrestris Greek organic mountain herb tea bio. (n.d.). Lelex Tea. lelextea.com/en/greek-organic-herbs-herbal-teas-mountain-tea/tribulus-terrestris-greek-organic-wild-mountain-herb-tea-bio

Turmeric black pepper tincture. (n.d.). Willamette Transplant. willamettetransplant.com/turmeric-black-pepper-tincture-diy-recipe/

Turmeric tea recipe. (n.d.). 101 Cookbooks. 101cookbooks.com/turmeric-tea/

12 cleansing herbs to help detoxify your body. (n.d.). Euphoric Herbals. euphoricherbals.com/blogs/blog/detox-herbs

The urinary tract & how it works. (n.d.). National Institute of Diabetes and Digestive and Kidney Diseases. niddk.nih.gov/health-information/urologic-diseases/urinary-tract-how-it-works

Vann, M. R. (2023, July 27). 4 natural remedies for nausea. Everyday Health. everydayhealth.com/digestive-health/natural-remedies-for-nausea/

Vickers, A., Zollman, C., & Lee, R. (2001). Herbal medicine. *Western Journal of Medicine*, *175*(2), 125–128. doi.org/10.1136/ewjm.175.2.125

Villines, Z. (2020, February 11). Can herbal remedies relieve endometriosis symptoms? Medical News Today. medicalnewstoday.com/articles/herbs-for-endometriosis

Visser, M. (2017, December 26). *14* must-have supplies for herbalists (plus a free printable herbal toolkit supply list). *Herbal Academy*. theherbalacademy.com/blog/supplies-for-herbalists/

Vitatree. (2023, March 10). Top 3 supplements you should never take with coffee. vitatree.com/blog/vitamind/vitaminb/magnesium/top-3-supplements-you-should-never-take-with-coffee

Wardle, C. (2023, September 6). Preventative vs proactive vs reactive care – What's the difference and why are they important? The Access Group. theaccessgroup.com/en-gb/blog/hsc-preventative-vs-proactive-vs-reactive-care-what-s-the-difference-and-why-are-they-important/

Watson, K. (2023, February 6). 30 natural ways to help treat polycystic ovary syndrome (PCOS). Healthline. healthline.com/health/womens-health/natural-treatment-pcos

WebMD Editorial Contributors. (n.d.-a). Herbs for endometriosis. WebMD. webmd.com/women/endometriosis/herbs-for-endometriosis

WebMD Editorial Contributors. (n.d.-b). Natural remedies to alleviate anxiety. WebMD. webmd.com/anxiety-panic/natural-remedies-for-anxiety

WebMD Editorial Contributors. (n.d.-c). Natural treatments for menopause symptoms. WebMD. webmd.com/menopause/menopause-natural-treatments

WebMD Editorial Contributors. (2023, September 5). 14 natural treatment tips for colds and flu. WebMD. webmd.com/cold-and-flu/14-tips-prevent-colds-flu-1

Welch, S. (2021, November 30). 9 herbs to relieve cold and flu symptoms. Farm and Dairy. farmanddairy.com/top-stories/9-herbs-to-relieve-cold-and-flu-symptoms/695280.html

Wells, K. (2021, April 28). *Sweet dreams sleep tincture recipe.* Wellness Mama. wellnessmama.com/remedies/sleep-tincture-recipe/

Wells, K. (2022, December 28). *Home remedies for pink eye.* Wellness Mama. wellnessmama.com/remedies/pink-eye/

West, H. (2024, January 19). 13 home remedies for constipation. Medical News Today. medicalnewstoday.com/articles/318694

What are pharmaceutical ointments? (n.d.). Vedantu. vedantu.com/biology/ointment

What does proactive medicine mean, and why should you be doing it? (2022, December 19). Biolite. biolitedubai.com/blog/what-does-proactive-medicine-mean-and-why-should-you-be-doing-it

What herbs are good for irritable bowel syndrome? (2021, May 20). Artigest IBS. artigestibs.co.za/our-stories/2021/5/20/what-herbs-are-good-for-irritable-bowel-syndrome

What is synergy - And why it matters. (2015, September 9). Gaia Herbs. gaiaherbs.com/blogs/seeds-of-knowledge/what-is-synergy-and-why-it-matters

What's the difference between herbal tea and a herbal infusion? (n.d.). Tiree Tea. tireetea.co.uk/whats-the-difference-between-herbal-tea-and-a-herbal-infusion/

Wiertsema, S. P., van Bergenhenegouwen, J., Garssen, J., & Knippels, L. M. J. (2021). The interplay between the gut microbiome and the immune system in the context of infectious diseases throughout life and the role of nutrition in optimizing treatment strategies. *Nutrients*, *13*(3), 886. doi.org/10.3390/nu13030886

Wiginton, K. (2023, July 26). Psoriasis treatments: How to get rid of psoriasis. WebMD. webmd.com/skin-problems-and-treatments/psoriasis/understanding-psoriasis-treatment

Wilde, M. (2010, August 14). *An early timeline of herbal medicine*. Monica Wilde Forager. monicawilde.com/an-early-timeline-of-herbal-medicine/

Wilde, M. (2021, July 3). Herbs and nutrition for vitiligo. *Napiers*. napiers.net/blogs/health-information/herbs-and-nutrition-for-vitiligo

Will. (n.d.). 6 simple homemade teas to boost your mood. The Gousto Blog. gousto.co.uk/blog/make-herbal-homemade-teas-from-scratch

Williams, N. (2021, August 23). Herbal versus synthetic medicines. News Medical. news-medical.net/health/Herbal-versus-Synthetic-Medicines.aspx

Wong, C. (2023a, February 5). Home remedies for poison ivy. Verywell Health. verywellhealth.com/natural-poison-ivy-remedies-89303

Wong, C. (2023b, March 22). 7 best herbs for memory and brain health. Verywell Mind. verywellmind.com/best-herbs-and-spices-for-brain-health-4047818

Wong, C. (2023c, October 19). 3 home remedies for burns that actually work. Verywell Health. verywellhealth.com/burn-remedies-89945

Wong, C. (2023d, October 24). 9 herbs to relieve menstrual cramps. Verywell Health. verywellhealth.com/herbs-for-menstrual-cramps-89901

Wong, C. (2024, March 6). 9 home remedies for varicose veins. Verywell Health. verywellhealth.com/natural-treatments-for-varicose-veins-89260

Wood betony. (n.d.). Peace Health. peacehealth.org/medical-topics/id/hn-3662000#hn-3662000-how-it-works

Wounds. (n.d.). Mount Sinai. mountsinai.org/health-library/condition/wounds

Yellow dock. (n.d.). Peace Health. peacehealth.org/medical-topics/id/hn-2189000#hn-2189000-how-it-works

Yohimbe bark (Corynanthe yohimbe). (n.d.). Kalustyan's. foodsofnations.com/products/yohimbe-bark

Made in the USA
Monee, IL
17 February 2025